Pass PACES:
essential study guide

D1355578

For Elsevier
Content Strategist: Pauline Graham
Content Development Specialist: Carole McMurray
Project Manager: Andrew Riley
Designer/Design Direction: Christian Bilbow

Pass PACES:
essential study guide

Edited by

Eirini Vasileiou Kasfiki, MB BCh MRCP FHEA PG Dip Med Ed

Ciaran WP Kelly, BA MB BCh (Hons) BAO MRCS

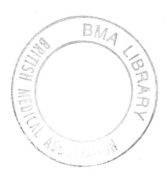

ELSEVIER

Edinburgh   London   New York   Oxford   Philadelphia   St Louis   Sydney   Toronto 2017

ELSEVIER

ISBN 978-0-7020-6845-4
eISBN 978-0-7020-6843-0

Notices
Knowledge and best practice in this field are constantly changing. As new research and experience broaden our understanding, changes in research methods, professional practices, or medical treatment may become necessary.

Practitioners and researchers must always rely on their own experience and knowledge in evaluating and using any information, methods, compounds, or experiments described herein. In using such information or methods they should be mindful of their own safety and the safety of others, including parties for whom they have a professional responsibility.

With respect to any drug or pharmaceutical products identified, readers are advised to check the most current information provided (i) on procedures featured or (ii) by the manufacturer of each product to be administered, to verify the recommended dose or formula, the method and duration of administration, and contraindications. It is the responsibility of practitioners, relying on their own experience and knowledge of their patients, to make diagnoses, to determine dosages and the best treatment for each individual patient, and to take all appropriate safety precautions.

To the fullest extent of the law, neither the Publisher nor the authors, contributors, or editors, assume any liability for any injury and/or damage to persons or property as a matter of products liability, negligence or otherwise, or from any use or operation of any methods, products, instructions, or ideas contained in the material herein.

your source for books, journals and multimedia in the health sciences

www.elsevierhealth.com

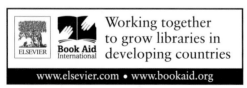

Working together to grow libraries in developing countries

www.elsevier.com • www.bookaid.org

The Publisher's policy is to use **paper manufactured from sustainable forests**

Printed in China

Contributors

Michael Crooks, MBChB (Hons), MD, MRCP
Jivendra Gosai, MBChB, BMSc(Hons), MRCP
Victoria Thorley-Dickinson, MBChB, MRC
Musab Elgaali, MBBS, MRCP
Anna Folwell, MBChb, MRCP

Contents

Station 5

Video Contents

Preface

Welcome to *Pass PACES: Essential Study Guide* for Your MRCP PACES Exam.

The exam consists of five 20-min stations. Stations 1 and 3 are the purely clinical stations with two patients in each station, Station 2 is the history-taking station, Station 4 is the communication and ethics station, with one patient or surrogate in each, and Station 5 is the new station for PACES exam, which has two patients.

Station 1
One respiratory case
One abdominal case or one renal case

Station 2
History-talking station

Station 3
One cardiology case
One neurology case

Station 4
Communication and ethics station

Station 5
Two brief consultation cases, where focused history and examination can be taken simultaneously

The PACES carousel can start with any of the above stations. Each candidate rotates from station to station, with 5 min between each station. Before entering clinical Stations 1 and 3, no preparation is required and the candidates have to wait for the examiners to let them enter the clinical stations. Before entering Stations 2, 4 and 5, though, these 5 min are valuable, as the description of the cases is given and adequate preparation is vital.

Stations 1 and 3

Each station consists of 20 min. There are two patients to be examined in each of these stations. That means you have 10 min with each patient. These 10 min are divided into:

- six minutes for patient examination and
- four minutes for presentation of your findings followed by questions by the examiners.

In these two stations (four cases), if your examination finishes prior to the 6 min you are given, examiners can start asking questions earlier (as soon as you have completed your examination). So it is very important that you take advantage of any minutes left to elicit any clinical findings, as you do not want to miss anything because you finished early.

Once the 6 min have passed, the examiners will stop your examination and start the 4 min of questioning.

The best way to find this balance of time for these stations is to time yourself when you practise for these stations. The more patients you practise the whole routine on without missing signs, the better prepared you will be to take full advantage of the 6 min given, and the more likely to finish on time, having found all the signs.

Stations 2 and 4 practically begin the moment you leave Stations 1 and 3. The 5-min break in between the stations is vital time prior to entering Stations 2 and 4. You will be given one scenario for each station, as well as paper and pencil to make preparation notes you think will be relevant. Take advantage of that and prepare for the cases you are going to face in the stations. More detail will be given in the following chapters. In each of these stations, apart from the 5-min preparation, you will get 20 min in the station. Your patient interaction time is 14 min with a 2-min warning from the examiners before your time is finished (i.e. after 12 min). Two minutes after the warning, the patient/surrogate will leave the room, and for the remaining 6 min of the station, you will get 1 min for reflection and 5 min for presentation of the case followed by questions from the examiners. If you finish your consultation before the allotted 14 min, you will have to stay silent in the room with the patient until the 14 min pass.

Station 5 starts as soon as Station 4 has finished, with 5 min of preparation outside the room, exactly as happens with Stations 2 and 4, but with one essential difference. Here you are given two cases to prepare and you do not know which one will be first when you enter the station. So, you have 5 min to prepare and take notes for two separate cases. Make sure you divide your time equally and adequately between the two. Upon entering the station, the examiners will show you the first case, and after 10 min you will be directed to the next case. Each case consists of 8 min of focused history and examination, followed by 2 min of examiners' questions. As with clinical Stations 1 and 3, if you finish your history and examination earlier than the 8 min given, examiners will start asking questions. Station 5 carries the most marks in the exam, so preparation for this station is vital (see chapter for further details).

The marking system is made up of a three-score system for each element examined in each station:

- Satisfactory: 2
- Borderline: 1
- Unsatisfactory: 0

The maximum score in PACES is 172 with an overall pass mark of 130. But scoring 130 is not the only requirement for passing the exam, as you also need to pass all the individual competencies assessed during the exam. That means that as well as achieving the pass mark of 130, you also need to meet the minimum score requirements for the clinical skills assessed:

A – physical examination: 14/24
B – identifying physical signs: 14/24
C – clinical communication: 10/16
D – differential diagnosis: 16/28
E – clinical judgment: 18/32
F – managing patient concerns: 10/16
G – maintaining patient welfare: 28/32

This book aims to help you with your preparation for the PACES exam and show you how to perform your best during the exam.

Throughout the book, you will find 'tip' boxes that contain helpful tips to help you with your preparation. They consist of important messages that we have identified that candidates are usually unaware of when they sit their exam for the first time. These boxes look like this:

> ### Tip!
> The best way to prepare for your PACES exam is to find a 'PACES buddy'. Match with a colleague who is at the same level of preparation as you and prepare together. Examine cases together, exchange roles of candidate/examiner and give feedback to each other. Try to aim at practising on two patients per day for the last 3 months prior to the real exam. Keep a record of the patients you see and the signs you come across so that you go back and read about each case.

Tip!

Do not forget to practise the nonclinical stations (Stations 2 and 4). Candidates usually underestimate them and give more importance to Stations 1 and 3; however, they are commonly failed stations, and it is easy to pass them so long as you have prepared well. Additionally you may get a difficult Station 1 patient, so preparing for Station 4 and achieving full marks there may save you from an overall 'fail', as you can compensate for lost marks.

The second type of box you will come across in this book are the 'mnemonic' boxes. They aim to give you lists of useful things in the exam that can be easily recalled when time is vital. They look like this:

MNEMONIC

How to pass PACES

'*PACES*'

Prepare with a friend

Assess each other on two

Cases per day for 3 months

Enjoy the preparation

Study the cases in this book

To help you with your preparation each of the clinical station chapters is accompanied with a podcast containing tips on how to approach the station in the examination room, and a video on the routine examination of each system, as it should be performed within the exam setting. The non clinical stations are accompanied by a video of a mock station that will help you understand the approach of the non clinical stations

The whole exam lasts 120 min, so take a deep breath, and before you know it, you will have finished it. Good luck and enjoy reading!

Eirini and Ciaran

Acknowledgements

We would like to thank the clinicians who helped with the book: Anoop Prakash, Sega Pathmanathan, John Smith and Tun Aung, as well as the technical team of Hull Institute of Learning and Simulation for their help with the interactive material: Makani Purva, Olivia Charlton, Chris Gay, Stuart Riby, Maggie Hutchinson and Matthew Graby.

We would also like to thank the patients who have helped us with the video production.

Respiratory

In most respiratory cases, the synopsis of the patient would be: 'This patient presents with shortness of breath. Please examine his respiratory system.'

Pulmonary fibrosis

Presenting a case of *pulmonary fibrosis*

Organize your presentation into the following categories:
1. Positive clinical findings and diagnosis
2. Presence of complications
3. Differential diagnosis
4. Workup.

> **Tip!**
> Pulmonary fibrosis is a very common case in PACES, so it is worth knowing inside out! The examiners will expect candidates to perform well, so for top marks your presentation must be excellent.

Positive clinical findings

General examination
- The patient may be breathless at rest; observe his respiratory rate and comment on the presence of oxygen.
- There may be peripheral cyanosis. Check for clubbing and signs of rheumatoid arthritis (RA) or connective tissue disease (CTD).

Chest examination
- Inspect the chest wall closely for scars suggestive of video-assisted thoracoscopic surgery (VATS) lung biopsy.
- Chest expansion may be reduced in severe disease.
- Percussion will be resonant.
- On auscultation, there will be bilateral, fine, end-crackles.

> **Tip!**
> Most commonly, your findings of fine crackles will be at the lung bases. If your patient has apical fibrosis, then it will impress the examiners if you mention possible differentials for apical fibrosis. Remember the mnemonic 'STARS'.

MNEMONIC

Apical fibrosis: *STARS*

*S*arcoidosis

*T*uberculosis (TB)

*A*nkylosing spondylitis, allergic bronchopulmonary aspergillosis (ABPA)

*R*adiation

*S*everal inhaled agents (extrinsic allergic alveolitis [EAA], silicosis, etc.)

Presence of complications

- Cor pulmonale:
  - Raised jugular venous pressure (JVP) and peripheral oedema.
- Pulmonary hypertension:
  - Raised JVP with giant V waves, right ventricular heave, peripheral oedema.

Differential diagnosis

- Left ventricular failure.
- Bronchiectasis – this is a common mistake in PACES – the character of the crackles and presence of wheeze and squeaks in bronchiectasis should help you differentiate.

CAUSES OF PULMONARY FIBROSIS: *VI$_2$CED ST*

*V*asculitides (Churg–Strauss, Wegener's)

*I*diopathic pulmonary fibrosis (IPF) and *I*nhaled agents

*C*onnective tissue disorders and rheumatological diseases

*E*osinophilic pneumonia

*D*rugs and radiation

*S*arcoidosis

*T*B

NB. The most common form is IPF and this should be mentioned first unless there are clear features of an underlying condition upon examination.

Workup

- Detailed history including features of CTD, occupation, environmental exposure, medications and family history.

- Blood tests including an autoimmune screen (anti-nuclear antibodies [ANA], extractable nuclear antigens [ENA], anti-neutrophil cytoplasmic antibodies [ANCA], rheumatoid factor [RF] and creatine kinase [CK]).
- Pulmonary function tests:
  - Spirometry, lung volumes and gas transfer (transfer factor for carbon monoxide).
- Chest X-ray (CXR).
- High-resolution computed tomography (HRCT) thorax.
- Referral to interstitial lung disease (ILD) multi-disciplinary team (MDT).

Model presentation

Mr Smith is a 65-year-old gentleman presenting with shortness of breath. On examination, he is short of breath at rest with a respiratory rate of 22. He has finger clubbing. On auscultation of his chest, he has bibasal, fine, end-inspiratory crackles. He has no evidence of cor pulmonale or CTD.

My findings are consistent with a diagnosis of IPF. My differential would include other causes of pulmonary fibrosis, which I would explore by taking a full detailed history with particular focus on features of CTD, occupational and environmental exposures, family history and drug history.

I would like to conclude my examination by obtaining bedside observations such as blood pressure, heart rate and oxygen saturations. I would like to arrange detailed pulmonary function tests and a CXR in the first instance.

If pulmonary function tests and CXR are consistent with pulmonary fibrosis, then I will arrange an HRCT thorax with subsequent discussion at the ILD MDT.

Discussion with the examiners

What investigations would you request for this patient?
- Blood tests:
  - Full blood count (FBC) may show polycythaemia in chronic hypoxia. Neutrophilia may be observed with infection or related to steroid therapy. Eosinophilia may suggest an alternative ILD (e.g. Churg–Strauss, eosinophilic pneumonia or drug reaction).
  - Urea and electrolytes (U&E) should be checked to assess for other organ involvement in CTD or vasculitis.
  - Autoimmune/CTD screen including RF, ANA, ENA, ANCA and CK.
  - Specific precipitins if EAA is suspected from the history or radiological features.

- Serum ACE may be elevated in sarcoidosis but is not particularly useful making a diagnosis.
- Pulmonary function tests:
  - Spirometry will demonstrate a restrictive pattern with reduced lung volumes and gas transfer.
- CXR:
  - The pattern will depend on the type of ILD.
  - IPF is associated with peripheral reticular shadowing predominately in lower zones.
- HRCT:
  - The pattern of HRCT changes will depend on the type of ILD.
  - IPF is associated with peripheral, basal and subpleural reticulation with or without honeycombing and little or no ground glass change.
- Invasive investigations:
  - Bronchoscopy for transbronchial biopsy or lavage is rarely necessary but can be useful in specific cases, for example, in sarcoidosis.
  - VATS lung biopsy is usually the best way to obtain histology in patients with ILD but is not necessary in patients with typical clinical and radiological features.

How would you manage this patient?

This will depend on the type of ILD – for the sake of this case, we describe the management of IPF.

- Supportive treatments form the mainstay of management, including breathlessness management techniques (opiates, fan therapy, etc.) and oxygen if hypoxic.
- Pirfenidone is a novel antifibrotic drug that slows the rate of lung function decline in IPF patients. It is licenced in the United Kingdom for patients with a forced vital capacity (FVC) of 50–80%.
- Nintedanib is a tyrosine kinase inhibitor that slows the rate of lung function decline in IPF patients. It is licenced in the United States, but not yet available in the United Kingdom for general use.
- Gastroesophageal reflux is prevalent in IPF and should be identified and treated.
- Prednisolone, azathioprine and N-acetylcysteine are no longer used, as this combination has been shown to be associated with increased mortality in IPF.

- High-dose methylprednisolone is still used in patients with acute exacerbations of IPF, but this is not evidence-based.
- IPF patients should be offered pulmonary rehabilitation.
- Lung transplant should be considered in younger patients with IPF.

What do you know about IPF?

- The most common fibrotic ILD
- More common in males than females
- Occurs in older patients (generally over 50 years of age; the average age at diagnosis is around 70)
- Poor prognosis with median survival around 3 years.

Name some drugs causing pulmonary fibrosis

- Methotrexate (look for signs of RA, also a cause of fibrosis!), amiodarone, cyclophosphamide, bleomycin, nitrofurantoin, sulphasalazine.

Do you know any other respiratory causes of finger clubbing?

- Lung cancer/mesothelioma
- Cystic fibrosis (CF) and non-CF bronchiectasis
- Empyema/lung abscess/TB.

Where to find respiratory cases for practise

The best places to find respiratory cases for exam practice are the respiratory ward, the acute medical unit and the respiratory clinics.

Pleural effusion

Presenting a case of a *pleural effusion*

Organize your presentation in the following four categories:

1. Positive clinical findings and diagnosis
2. Causes for pleural effusion
3. Investigations
4. Treatment.

> **Tip!**
> As with all respiratory cases, present your findings in the order in which you identified them: general inspection from the bedside, hands, face, neck, peripheries, and then focus on to the main finding of pleural effusion.

Positive clinical findings

General examination

- The patient may be breathless at rest; observe the respiratory rate and assess chest expansion from the end of the bed.
- Look for finger clubbing and nicotine staining that will raise your suspicion of malignant pleural disease.
- The patient may have features of rheumatological disease, suggesting this as an underlying cause for their effusion.
- The trachea may be deviated away from a large effusion.
- The presence of lymphadenopathy will point to malignancy.
- Observe the JVP for signs of fluid overload, raising the possibility of heart failure as a cause for pleural effusion.

Chest examination

- Carefully inspect the chest for signs of previous pleural intervention (dressings over aspiration sites and scars from drains and/or thoracic surgery).
- Formally assess chest expansion to confirm your earlier observation from the end of the bed (expansion is reduced on the side of the effusion).
- Percussion will reveal the classical stony-dullness of a pleural effusion.
- On auscultation, there will be reduced breath sounds and reduced vocal resonance over the effusion. You may notice bronchial breathing immediately above the level of the effusion.
- If you choose to undertake tactile vocal fremitus, this will be reduced over the effusion.

Tip!

Although there are multiple diseases that can cause pleural effusion, you cannot cover all of them in your presentation. It is important, however, to comment on the presence or absence of findings that would point toward a specific cause. For example, after presenting a pleural effusion, you can demonstrate you have considered underlying causes by mentioning the presence or absence of signs of heart failure or CTD, etc.

Workup

- Detailed history including onset of symptoms and associated features, occupational history (i.e., asbestos exposure), social history including smoking status and drug history.
- Blood tests (look for signs of underlying infection, hepatic, renal or CTD).
- CXR.
- Diagnostic pleural aspiration under ultrasound guidance.
- Contrast computed tomography (CT) thorax (if diagnosis remains unclear, following pleural aspiration).
- VATS with pleural biopsy if diagnosis remains unclear following above investigations.

Treatment

- Supplementary oxygen if required.
- Therapeutic aspiration or intercostal chest drain insertion:
  - The most appropriate intervention will depend on the clinical circumstances.
- Treat the underlying cause.

Model presentation

This patient, who presented with breathlessness, is comfortable at rest with no supplemental oxygen.

He does not have finger clubbing or cyanosis, and his trachea is central. There is no cervical lymphadenopathy. On examination of his chest, expansion is reduced on the left side, the percussion note is stony-dull over the left base and tactile vocal fremitus is also reduced over the same area. The breath sounds are diminished in this area, with an area of bronchial breathing above that.

In summary, this patient's breathlessness is due to a left-sided pleural effusion. I have not identified any signs that would suggest an underlying cause for a pleural effusion in this patient. Specifically, the JVP is not raised, there is no peripheral oedema to suggest heart failure, and there is no clubbing, cervical lymphadenopathy or cachexia to suggest malignancy.

I would like to finish my examination by looking at the observation and temperature chart. I would like to take a full history, including occupation, smoking and drug histories.

Tip!

Be aware that dullness over an area does not necessarily mean pleural effusion! You have to put all the other signs together, as the differential diagnosis of a dull lung base is broad:

1. Pleural effusion
2. Collapse
3. Consolidation
4. Pleural thickening
5. Raised hemidiaphragm

Discussion with the examiners

What are the possible causes of pleural effusion?

Unilateral effusions are usually (but not always) exudates, and the most common causes for exudates are:

- malignancy (carcinoma of the lung, mesothelioma, lymphoma, metastatic malignancy from distant primary)
- parapneumonic
- TB
- autoimmune/CTD (RA, systemic lupus erythematosus)
- pancreatitis
- pulmonary embolism
- benign asbestos effusion
- post-myocardial infarction syndrome
- post-coronary artery bypass surgery
- drugs; and
- yellow nail syndrome (rare).

MNEMONIC

Most common exudates: *MIC*

*M*alignancy
*I*nfections
*C*onnective tissue disease

Bilateral pleural effusions are usually transudates. The following cause transudate effusions:

- Congestive cardiac failure
- Liver cirrhosis
- Hypoalbuminaemia
- Renal failure, nephrotic syndrome, peritoneal dialysis
- Hypothyroidism
- Constrictive pericarditis
- Mitral stenosis
- Meigs' syndrome.

MNEMONIC

Bilateral pleural effusion:

All the failures

Renal, liver, cardiac and thyroid

Would you perform a diagnostic aspiration?

If the clinical picture leads you to suspect a transudate, then the cause should be treated and you should only investigate further if the effusion persists.

What tests would you send the pleural fluid for?

- Pleural aspiration and analysis of pleural fluid for:
  - pH (In the presence of pneumonia, a pH <7.2 is suggestive of a complex parapneumonic effusion or empyema and a chest drain is indicated; a low pH can also be seen in malignancy and in this setting is associated with a poor prognosis.)
  - biochemistry:
    - protein and LDH (comparison with serum protein and LDH for differentiating exudates from transudates using Light's criteria)
    - glucose (very low levels are seen in RA)
    - amylase (specific cases only)
    - cholesterol and triglycerides (specific cases only)

- microbiology and
  - gram stain and acid-fast bacilli stain
  - bacterial and mycobacterial cultures
- cytology (60% of malignant pleural effusions can be diagnosed by fluid analysis alone).

What are the Light's criteria of an exudate?

One of the following should be fulfiled for the effusion to be characterized as an exudate:

- Pleural fluid protein/serum protein >0.5.
- Pleural fluid LDH/serum LDH >0.6.
- Pleural fluid LDH >2/3 of the upper limit of serum LDH.

What other investigations would you request for this patient?

- Blood tests:
  - FBC
  - Biochemical profile (BCP), protein
  - LDH
  - Autoimmune screen
  - B-type Natriuretic Peptide
  - Blood cultures.
- Other tests depending on the initial suspicion and the success of the previous test to reveal a diagnosis:
  - CT with contrast
  - Computed tomography pulmonary arteriography
  - Pleural biopsy:
    - VATS
    - CT guided in some cases.

How would you manage this patient?

The treatment will depend on the underlying cause, the patient's clinical status and patient preference.

In asymptomatic patients with an effusion of known cause, it may be appropriate to simply observe.

Patients who are symptomatic may require drainage of the effusion either by means of therapeutic aspiration or intercostal chest drain insertion.

Management of malignant pleural effusions will depend on the patients prognosis:

- If prognosis is very limited, then therapeutic aspiration alone may be appropriate.
- If prognosis is good, then a more definitive approach is warranted:
  - Intercostal chest drain insertion and pleurodesis.
  - Medical or surgical thoracoscopy with pleurodesis.
  - Indwelling pleural catheter insertion.

What are the indications for chest drain in parapneumonic effusions?
- Purulent or turbid, cloudy fluid.
- Presence of gram-stained organisms in the pleural fluid.
- Pleural fluid pH <7.2.
- Persistent infection and effusion, despite correct antibiotic treatment.
- Symptomatic big pleural effusions.

MNEMONIC

Indications for chest drain in parapneumonic effusions: *PIGS 7.2*

*P*urulent fluid (empyema)
*I*nfection persists
*G*ram stain
*S*ymptomatic
<7.2 pH

Bronchiectasis

Tip!

After scanning the room, check the patient's breathing. Stand at the end of the bed and observe the patient at rest to assess their respiratory rate and breathing pattern. Observe both inspiratory and expiratory phases (patients with airflow obstruction may have prolonged expiration). Then ask the patient to take a deep breath to emphasize any asymmetry in chest expansion.

> **Tip!**
> Before examining a patient in the respiratory station, spend a few seconds looking around the room for clues to the diagnosis (oxygen, inhalers, sputum pots). In a case of bronchiectasis, the clue would be a sputum pot. If you see a sputum pot, ask the patient to cough. In bronchiectasis, the cough will probably be productive.

Presenting a case of *bronchiectasis*

Organize your presentation into the following categories:
1. Positive clinical findings and diagnosis
2. Presence of complications
3. Differential diagnosis
4. Workup.

> **Tip!**
> As with all respiratory cases, present your findings in the order you identified them: general inspection from the bedside, hands, face, neck, peripheries, and then focus on to the main finding of bronchiectasis.

Positive clinical findings

General examination

- The patient may be breathless at rest and if they cough during the consultation, it may sound wet. Look for sputum pots.
- On examination of the hands, there may or may not be finger clubbing.
- If the patient has had previous lung resection for localized bronchiectasis, you may observe asymmetrical chest expansion from the end of the bed and on palpation of the neck, the trachea will be deviated toward the side of the surgery.
- As with most chronic respiratory diseases, bronchiectasis can result in chronic respiratory failure leading to pulmonary hypertension and cor pulmonale.

Chest examination

- Inspect carefully for scars suggestive of resection of localized disease.
- Chest expansion will depend on disease distribution and whether patient has had previous lung surgery.

- Auscultation of the chest may reveal mixed inspiratory and expiratory coarse crackles, occasional squeaks that change character after coughing and wheeze that can be focal or widespread.

Presence of complications

Before finishing your presentation, comment on signs of pulmonary hypertension and cor pulmonale.

The following clinical signs suggest pulmonary hypertension and cor pulmonale:

- Raised JVP with tall V waves
- Left parasternal heave
- Loud P2 component of second heart sound
- Peripheral oedema (pedal oedema/sacral oedema).

Differential diagnosis

The differential diagnosis will depend on the clinical findings; however, a common area of confusion in PACES is differentiating the crackles of ILD/pulmonary fibrosis and bronchiectasis. There is no substitute for experience and therefore practice makes perfect, but take the following into account:

- Finger clubbing can be present in both conditions.
- Fibrosis typically causes 'velcro-like' crackles, whereas the crackles in bronchiectasis are coarser.
- Evidence of airflow obstruction (prolonged expiratory phase of respiration and wheeze) should point you toward bronchiectasis rather than fibrosis.

Workup

- Spirometry (usually an obstructive picture: forced expiratory volume in 1 s (FEV_1)/FVC <0.7).
- CXR.
- HRCT (gold standard for the diagnosis).
- Blood tests (identifying the underlying cause) and sputum cultures (to identify colonizing organisms and pathogens of exacerbations).

Model presentation

This patient who presents with shortness of breath is not breathless at rest, but has a cough productive of large amounts of (mucoid/purulent) sputum, as evident by the sputum pot on the table. On examination, there is finger clubbing but no peripheral or central cyanosis. His chest expansion is reduced but symmetrical, the percussion note is resonant, and on auscultation, there are widespread inspiratory and expiratory crepitations, which alter with coughing. There are also occasional squeaks and mild widespread expiratory wheeze.

In summary, this patient's clinical findings are consistent with bronchiectasis. There are no signs of secondary pulmonary hypertension.

I would like to conclude my examination by looking at the observation chart and performing bedside spirometry.

For further assessment, I would like to take further history, including smoking, past medical and family histories.

I would then like to request investigations in the forms of CXR, spirometry and blood tests. The patient will need an HRCT of his chest to confirm the diagnosis.

> **Tip!**
>
> When diagnosing a case of bronchiectasis, you are unlikely to be able to confirm an underlying aetiology from your examination in PACES apart from certain specific cases. If you have not been able to identify a cause, do not worry; this may form part of subsequent discussion with the examiners. If you identify any of the signs below, you should include them in your presentation:
>
> Yellow nails and lymphoedema: suspect yellow nail syndrome
> Right-sided heart sounds on auscultation: Kartagener's syndrome
> Finger pinpricks in young suggesting diabetes: CF
> Focal bronchiectasis: bronchial obstruction

Discussion with the examiners

What are the causes of bronchiectasis?
- Autoimmune (RA, inflammatory bowel disease).
- ABPA.
- Anatomical and mucociliary defects (primary ciliary dyskinesia, Kartagener's syndrome CF, young syndrome, yellow nail syndrome).
- Anatomical obstruction of the bronchi (tumours, foreign bodies).
- Immunodeficiency.

- Infections (human immunodeficiency virus, TB, respiratory childhood infections).
- Idiopathic.

> **MNEMONIC**
>
> **Causes of bronchiectasis: $(AI)_3$**
>
> **A**utoimmune
> **A**BPA
> **A**natomical and mucociliary defects of focal obstruction
> **I**nfections
> **I**mmunodeficiency
> **I**diopathic

What investigations would you like to perform for this patient?
- Spirometry (will usually demonstrate an obstructive pattern, but can be mixed).
- CXR.
- HRCT will confirm the diagnosis and assess the distribution of disease.
- Blood tests (immunoglobulins, aspergillus serology).
- Specialist tests if a specific underlying disease is suspected (sweat chloride test for CF).
- Sputum for bacterial and mycobacterial culture.

What is the treatment for bronchiectasis?
- Regular physiotherapy for airway clearance is the cornerstone of bronchiectasis treatment.
- Treat the underlying cause if possible (steroids and antifungals in ABPA, preventing aspiration in recurrent aspiration-related bronchiectasis, immunoglobulins in patients with specific deficiencies).
- Treat infective exacerbations promptly (targeted antibiotic therapy).
- Smoking cessation.
- Vaccination.
- Surgery in selected cases (lobectomy/pneumonectomy in localized bronchiectasis, and massive haemoptysis, lung transplant).

How is CF diagnosed?

- Clinical suspicion.
- Sweat chloride test.
- DNA testing for known mutations (most common mutation is ΔF508 mutation in chromosome 7, which encodes the cystic fibrosis transmembrane conductance regulator protein).

What are the systems that are affected by CF?

- Respiratory system (bronchiectasis, recurrent infections, sinus problems).
- Gastrointestinal system (pancreatic insufficiency, bowel obstruction, diabetes, biliary cirrhosis, rectal prolapse, malabsorption).
- Genitourinary system (reduced fertility or infertility).

What is yellow nail syndrome?

Rare medical condition with the combination of lymphoedema, yellow dystrophic nails, bronchiectasis and pleural effusions.

What is Kartagener's syndrome?

It is the combination of situs inversus combined with primary ciliary dyskinesia and can lead to bronchiectasis.

Lobectomy/pneumonectomy

Presenting a case of a *lobectomy/pneumonectomy*

You should organize your presentation into the following categories:

1. Positive clinical findings and diagnosis.
2. Features on examination (if present) that point to an indication for lobectomy/pneumonectomy.
3. Workup with relation to the provided clinical scenario.

> **Tip!**
> If you follow the routine that should be applied to all respiratory cases described previously, you should notice both the surgical scar and the asymmetry of chest expansion on general inspection of the patient. That will make you suspect lobectomy or pneumonectomy before formally examining the patient.

Positive clinical findings

Your presentation should follow the findings in the order in which you discovered them.

General examination
- The patient may be breathless at rest. Fully expose the patient's chest and ask him to take a deep breath while you observe from the end of the bed. You will notice reduced expansion on the side of the lung resection.
- The patient may have finger clubbing, suggesting the possibility of bronchiectasis, abscess or malignancy as causes for lung resection.
- The patient's trachea will be deviated toward the side of the resection, suggesting loss of lung volume on this side.
- A detailed general examination should be undertaken to look for associated conditions providing clues to the reason for lung resection.

Chest examination
- On inspection, you will notice reduced expansion on the side of the lung resection. Surgical scars will be visible. This will usually be a thoracotomy scar, but VATS is increasingly being used for lung resections and therefore it is very important you undertake close inspection of the chest wall including in the axillae.
- You will notice reduced expansion on formal assessment with dullness to percussion at the site of resection.
- On auscultation, breath sounds will be diminished over the resected portion of lung, but be aware transmitted breath sounds are often audible and can confuse matters; therefore, identification of the scar and other features are crucial and will guide you. Pay attention to other sounds that point toward an indication for lung resection; for example, squeaks, wheeze and coarse crackles are indicative of bronchiectasis.

Workup

Your suggested workup will depend on the brief scenario provided in the station. It is likely to include:
- detailed history with particular reference to details of the lung surgery, including the indication and preresection lung function
- blood tests (only if appropriate to the clinical scenario)
- pulmonary function tests
- CXR; and

- CT thorax (if you are considering surgical complications or recurrence of malignancy, a contrast CT thorax would be appropriate; if you are considering bronchiectasis, then an HRCT thorax would be appropriate; a CXR would normally be undertaken before progressing to CT).

Model presentation

This patient, who presented with breathlessness, is comfortable at rest. His trachea is deviated to the right side. On examination of his chest, he has a right-sided thoracotomy scar with reduced chest expansion, dull percussion note and absent breath sounds also on the right side. Examination of the left lung field was unremarkable.

In summary, this patient has had a pneumonectomy in the past. I did not identify any physical signs to suggest the underlying condition requiring surgery; however, possible indications for pneumonectomy include malignancy, TB and complicated bronchiectasis. His presentation with breathlessness could be related to the initial indication for pneumonectomy or a new pathology.

I would like to look at his observation chart and take a more detailed history, particularly focusing on his respiratory symptoms and thorough past medical and smoking histories.

Tip!

If the trachea is not deviated to the scar site, and the breath sounds are normal on the scar side, whereas you can identify abnormal breathing sounds on the other side, consider single lung transplant.

Discussion with the examiners

What are the indications for pneumonectomy?
- Bronchiectasis
- TB
- Malignancy.

What are the reasons for lobectomy?
- Bronchiectasis
- Lung abscess
- TB

- Solitary pulmonary nodule – suspected malignancy
- Confirmed malignancy.

Chronic obstructive pulmonary disease

Presenting a case of *chronic obstructive pulmonary disease (COPD)*

Organize your presentation into the following categories:
1. Positive clinical findings and diagnosis
2. Presence of complications
3. Differential diagnosis
4. Workup.

Positive clinical findings

Present the positive findings in the order in which you have identified them.

General examination
- The patient may be breathless at rest with audible wheeze. Look for inhalers next to the bed or use of oxygen therapy. Observe the patient's breathing from the end of the bed and note the respiratory rate and pattern. You may notice a prolonged expiratory phase during respiration, suggestive of airflow obstruction.
- On examining the patient's hands, you may notice nicotine staining. You should assess for hypercapnia by observing for a flapping tremor with the patient's arms outstretched, wrists cocked back and fingers apart.
- On examining the patient's neck, you may see an elevated JVP if the patient has secondary pulmonary hypertension and cor pulmonale. The patient's trachea will be central and there should not normally be any palpable lymphadenopathy.

Chest examination
- On inspection, you may notice the use of accessory muscles of respiration, recession of the lower intercostal muscles on inspiration and/or pursed-lip breathing. You should look carefully for scars suggestive of lung resection to treat lung cancer or lung volume reduction surgery.
- The chest will be hyperinflated, resulting in symmetrically reduced chest expansion.

- On percussion, you may note symmetrical hyperresonance with loss of dullness over the heart.
- Auscultation of the chest will reveal quiet breath sounds with widespread expiratory wheeze. You may also notice a prolonged expiratory phase of respiration during auscultation.

Presence of complications

Pulmonary hypertension or cor pulmonale signs (raised JVP with giant V waves, loud P2 component of the second heart sound, parasternal heaves or thrills, peripheral oedema).

Differential diagnosis

Your differential diagnosis will depend on the positive findings on examination. Do not feel obliged to provide an exhaustive differential diagnosis list. You must be able to justify each differential diagnosis based on your findings.

Workup

- Detailed history with particular reference to smoking history, occupation history (coal mining and biomass workers), family history (α1-antitrypsin).
- Spirometry (obstructive pattern – FEV1/FVC <0.7).
- CXR.
- Arterial blood gas (ABG).
- Blood tests (this will depend on the clinical scenario – blood tests do not have a role in the diagnosis of COPD unless α1-antitrypsin deficiency is suspected).

Model presentation

This patient, who presented with shortness of breath and cough is breathless at rest, with audible wheeze heard from the end of the bed. I can see a salbutamol inhaler by his bedside.

On examination of his hands, there are nicotine stains, but no finger clubbing or peripheral cyanosis.

There is no palpable cervical lymphadenopathy.

On inspection, the patient is using accessory muscles of respiration and there is recession of the lower intercostal muscles during inspiration. His expiration is prolonged with a reversed ratio of inspiration/expiration time, and he is pursing his lips while breathing.

Chest expansion is equal on both sides, but is primarily vertical, with reduced horizontal expansion. The percussion note is hyperresonant over both lung fields.

On auscultation of his chest, the breath sounds are slightly diminished, and there is widespread expiratory wheeze.

There is no peripheral oedema, the JVP is not raised and heart sounds are normal.

In summary this patient has evidence of chronic obstructive pulmonary disease, with no signs of cor pulmonale.

I would like to finish my examination by looking at the observation and temperature chart and performing spirometry to confirm airflow obstruction.

Discussion with the examiners

What investigations would you want for this patient?

- FBC (neutrophilia due to infection or steroids, polycythaemia secondary to chronic hypoxia).
- BCP and C-reactive protein (CRP):
  - α1-antitrypsin assay (if young/nonsmoker).
  - CXR (hyperinflation, bullae, pneumothorax, consolidation, flat hemidiaphragms, large central pulmonary arteries, oligaemic lung fields).
  - ECG.
  - ABG (type 1 or type 2 respiratory failure).
  - Sputum for microscopy, culture and sensitivity.
  - Lung function tests (spirometry is important to demonstrate airflow obstruction, but measurement of lung volumes and gas transfer can provide additional information).
- HRCT is the most sensitive test to diagnose emphysema.

Diagnosis: post-bronchodilator spirometry demonstrates airflow obstruction = FEV1/FVC <0.7.

What are the most common pathogens to cause infective exacerbations in COPD patients?

- *Haemophilus influenza*
- *Streptococcus pneumonia*
- *Moraxella catarrhalis.*

How do you classify the severity of COPD?

With FEV1 measurement against predicted values:

- FEV1 >80% mild
- FEV1 50–79% moderate
- FEV1 30–49% severe
- FEV1 <30% very severe.

How do you treat stable COPD?

Step 1:

- Short-acting β2 agonist or short-acting muscarinic antagonist as required.

Step 2:

- If FEV1 >50%: regular long-acting β2 agonist or long-acting muscarinic antagonist.
- If FEV1 <50%: regular combined inhaled corticosteroid and long-acting β2 agonist, or long-acting muscarinic antagonist.

Step 3:

- Long-acting muscarinic antagonist and combined inhaled corticosteroid and long-acting β2 agonist.

Other treatments

- Smoking cessation
- Annual flu vaccination
- Pneumonococcal vaccination
- Consider oral theophylline if inhalers are not working
- Consider furosemide in cor pulmonale
- Consider long-term oxygen therapy (LTOT) in patients who meet the criteria.

When is LTOT indicated?

LTOT refers to the use of oxygen for >15 h per day with the aim of prolonging the life of the patient with COPD:

- Patients should be encouraged to stop smoking and if they fail to do so, a formal risk assessment should be performed and they should be educated about the risk of fire.
- In some centres, smoking is deemed an absolute contraindication to home oxygen therapy; however, other centres are more lenient.

- ABG criteria (two samples should be taken at least 3 weeks apart when symptoms are stable):
  - if PO2 <7.3
  - if PO2 = 7.3–8, but the patient has:
    - signs of cor pulmonale
    - secondary polycythaemia; and
    - nocturnal hypoxia.

Abdomen

In most abdominal cases, the synopsis of the patient would be: 'This patient presents with abdominal pain. Please examine.'

Chronic liver disease

Presenting a case of *chronic liver disease*

> **Tip!**
> Most findings in a case like this are elicited just by inspection. The best way to present in this station is to mention the positive findings in the same order as you discovered them in your examination. Presentation of your findings in this way will lead you to your final diagnosis in any case at the abdominal station. In this station, avoid mentioning negative findings.

Positive clinical findings

Comment specifically on the relevant findings below, if present:

General inspection: malnourished, icteric (jaundiced), cachectic patient, clubbing, leuconychia, Dupuytren's contracture, palmar erythema, spider naevi, gynaecomastia, loss of muscle mass, loss of body hair, petechiae, ecchymosis, parotid gland enlargement. Comment on each of these findings, if present, as you notice them.

When you have finished presentation of your inspection findings, concentrate on the *abdominal findings*:

- Abdominal distention
- Caput medusa
- Hepatomegaly (comment on shape, size, consistency and the existence of tenderness of the liver edge)
- Ascites.

Finish your identified signs with any *visible scars* on the abdomen (ascetic paracentesis, liver biopsy or liver transplant, presented in different chapter).

> **Tip!**
> To achieve full marks for your presentation, after presenting a diagnosis of chronic liver disease (CLD), you should comment on:
> - whether the disease is compensated or decompensated and
> - possible clues from your examination that may reveal the underlying aetiology for this patient's disease.

Findings that would lead you to identify a possible aetiology for the patient's diagnosis of CLD can be elicited from your inspection findings. For example, if the patient is a middle-aged female and you find xanthelasmata and excoriation marks on examination, then primary biliary cirrhosis should be your top differential, but if the patient has evidence of diabetes, for example, needle marks on the fingertips and with bronze skin, then haemochromatosis should be top of the list. In the past, the presence of tattoos may have been presented in the PACES exam as a possible clue for viral hepatitis. It is best if you avoid such a connection, but you can comment on the existence of tattoos as a general finding. Kayser–Fleischer rings in the iris will make you suspect Wilson's disease. If no clues are identified from the examination as to the aetiology of the cirrhosis, just present your differentials with the most common at the top.

MNEMONIC

Signs of decompensation of CLD: *JASE* (and how to check for them)

*J*aundice (skin and sclera)
*A*scites (abdominal distension, fluid wave, shifting dullness)
*S*plenomegaly/caput medusa
*E*ncephalopathy (make sure you check for hepatic flap)

Workup

- Detailed history, including travel and social history
- Full blood count (FBC), urea and electrolytes, liver function tests (LFTs), clotting screen
- Full liver screen
- Abdominal ultrasound
- Endoscopy.

Model presentation

This patient, who presents with episodes of haematemesis, looks cachectic on general inspection. On closer inspection, he has signs of malnutrition, such as leuconychia and loss of muscle mass in his limbs, and stigmata of CLD, namely palmar erythema, multiple spider naevi and jaundice.

His abdomen looks distended and there is shifting dullness, evidence of at least moderate ascites. On palpation of his abdomen, there is hepatomegaly, with no tender liver edge, 5 cm below the costal margin. He also has spleno-megaly, with the spleen being just above the umbilicus.

There is no hepatic tremor in his outstretched hands, but I could not formally test for encephalopathy, as I did not have the opportunity to talk with the patient.

In summary, the diagnosis for this patient is CLD, which is decompensated at the moment, evident by the presence of ascites, jaundice and splenomegaly.

I could not elicit from the clinical examination what the cause for his CLD might be.

The episodes of haematemesis are most likely related to portal hypertension, and I would like to admit this patient to hospital for further investigation.

I would like to finish my examination by performing a full set of observations and urinalysis. I would also like to take a more detailed history from the patient, specifically travel, family and social histories, to help identify a cause for his liver disease.

I would then proceed on a full liver screen and an ultrasound scan (USS) of the abdomen, and depending on his haemodynamic stability and the presence of other episodes of haematemesis, he may need an oesophago-gastro-duodenoscopy (OGD) during this inpatient episode.

Discussion with the examiners

Possible questions that may be asked by the examiners in this case, if not already presented, are:

What are the consequences of CLD?
- Portal hypertension and variceal/upper gastrointestinal bleed.
- Liver dysfunction and failure, failure of protein production, coagulopathy and encephalopathy.
- Infection of developed ascites (spontaneous bacterial peritonitis [SBP]).
- Cancer (hepatocellular carcinoma).

What are the causes of decompensation?
- Electrolyte imbalances
- Bleeding
- Infection
- Drugs and alcohol
- Constipation.

What are the causes of CLD?

The most common cause of CLD in the United Kingdom is alcoholic liver disease. Other common causes in developed countries are chronic viral hepatitis (B, C), haemochromatosis and nonalcoholic liver disease. Rarer causes are autoimmune hepatitis, primary biliary sclerosis, primary sclerosing cholangitis, Wilson's disease, α-1 antitrypsin deficiency, drugs, granulomatous liver disease, polycystic liver disease, nonviral hepatic infections and veno-occlusive disease.

MNEMONIC

Causes of CLD: *MAN-DIVA*

Metabolic causes, e.g. Wilson's, haemochromatosis, α-1 antitrypsin deficiency

Alcohol

Nonalcoholic fatty liver disease

Drugs, e.g. phenytoin, isoniazide, methotrexate

Infections, e.g. bacterial (*Staphylococcus aureus*)/parasitic (amoebiasis, hydatid disease)

Viral hepatitis, e.g. hepatitis B and C

Autoimmune causes, e.g. autoimmune hepatitis, primary biliary cirrhosis, primary sclerosing cholangitis

---

How do you interpret the caput medusa finding?

The abdominal wall veins drain in the iliofemoral system (lower) and the thoracic wall (upper). When portal hypertension develops, the umbilical vein opens and blood from the portal venous system flows through it toward the abdominal wall veins. To check whether prominent abdominal veins in the abdominal wall are caput medusa secondary to portal hypertension, block with your hand the dilated veins below the umbilicus, and determine the direction they fill when you relieve the pressure. In portal-systemic hypertension, blood should be directed away from the umbilicus.

Investigations

What investigations would you request for this patient?

Blood tests:

- LFTs
- Clotting screen (reflects the degree of hepatic synthetic dysfunction)
- γ-Glutamyl transferase (typically higher in alcoholic liver disease)

- Biochemical profile (hyponatraemia due to secondary hypoaldosteronism, renal failure due to hepatorenal syndrome)
- FBC (macrocytic anaemia, thrombocytopenia)
- Full liver screen to identify possible cause:
  - Iron studies with ferritin, total iron binding capacity
  - Hepatitis serology
  - Immunoglobulins
  - Autoantibodies
  - α-Feto-protein (AFP)
  - Ceruloplasmin
  - α-1 Antitrypsin levels.

Other tests that should be performed:

- Liver ultrasound with Doppler studies will demonstrate hepatomegaly, splenomegaly, focal liver lesions, hepatic vein thrombosis and reversed flow in the portal vein, and ascites.
- Ascitic tap with fluid sent for urgent microbiology, biochemistry and cultures; a WCC >250 cells/μL indicates SBP.
- Liver biopsy may be needed to confirm the diagnosis (and is the gold standard for diagnosis of cirrhosis but is not required if clinical examination and noninvasive investigations have already provided a diagnosis).

What are the complications of CLD?

MNEMONIC

Main complications of CLD: *ABCDE-ST*

Ascites
Bleeding (variceal)
Carcinoma (hepatocellular)
Different organ involvement (hepatorenal syndrome)
Encephalopathy
Spontaneous bacterial peritonitis
Thrombosis of the portal vein

How would you manage this patient?

This patient's treatment should be targeted toward both the acute presentation of variceal bleeding and the underlying diagnosis of CLD.

Variceal bleed

- If the patient was haemodynamically unstable, initial resuscitation measures are required, including:
  - Fluid resuscitation
  - Prophylactic antibiotics prior to endoscopy
  - Terlipressin
  - Proton pump inhibitor infusion
  - Transfusion of blood products; and
  - Correction of anticoagulation.
- Definitive treatment by urgent endoscopy for ligation/sclerotherapy of varices is the priority.

Chronic liver disease

The targets for the management of cirrhotic patients are:
- Identifying and treating the underlying pathology (e.g. if alcoholic liver disease is the diagnosis, abstinence from alcohol is essential).
- Screening for hepatocellular carcinoma:
  - Patients with CLD are, in general, at higher risk of developing hepatocellular carcinoma (HCC), and thus liver ultrasound with AFP measurement should be performed at regular intervals.
- Controlling variceal bleeding:
  - Confirmed varices warrant prophylactic treatment for prevention of further bleeding, which is usually in the form of nonselective beta blockers (propranolol) or combined with endoscopic treatment (ligation/sclerotherapy).
- Managing ascites:
  - Spironolactone and salt restriction are the initial treatments of choice, with the addition of furosemide when further diuresis is needed or hyperkalemia is an issue.
- Avoiding liver and renal toxins: all current medications will need to be optimized so the patient does not further deteriorate
- Provide nutritional support with supplementary vitamins and dietician involvement
- Treat acute complications and:
  - Patients who present with acute complications of their disease, such as SBP, or acute electrolyte derangement, will of course need to receive targeted treatment accordingly.

- Depending on multiple factors, including the underlying cause of the cirrhosis, patient may be a candidate for liver transplantation.

What predictive models do you know for determining the prognosis in CLD?

The most commonly used model is Child–Pugh classification:

Parameter	Points		
	1	2	3
Ascites	No	Mild	Moderate
Albumin	>35	28–35	<28
PT times the control	<4	4–6	>6
INR	<1.7	1.7–2.3	>2.3
Encephalopathy	None	Mild	Moderate
Bilirubin	Normal	34–50	>50

Class A (<6 points), Class B (7–9 points) and Class C (10–15 points).

Another model used is the MELD score (model of end-stage liver disease), especially for possible candidates for liver transplant, which takes into account bilirubin levels, creatinine levels, aetiology of the diagnosis and INR.

Different stages of CLD will predict different prognoses for patients; however, in the PACES examination, you will not be asked minute details of the scoring systems. Just mentioning the two classification systems will be enough for you to achieve full marks in this station.

Where to find abdominal cases to practise

You should pay a visit to gastroenterology wards, hepatology clinics, as well as haematology clinics and haematology wards of your hospital.

Hepatomegaly

Presenting a case of *hepatomegaly*

If your examination findings are consistent with CLD, then present the case accordingly (see the CLD case). If, however, you find hepatomegaly but cannot identify any stigmata of CLD, then start your presentation with your main finding of hepatomegaly, and then move on to important negative or important positive findings that will help you to make a diagnosis.

Positive clinical findings

Start your presentation with a detailed description of the finding of hepatomegaly, commenting on size, consistency and tenderness of the liver edge.

> **Tip!**
> If your main finding is hepatomegaly, after presenting the finding, make sure to mention important negative or positive findings. That will show the examiners that you have a list of possible differential diagnoses for this clinical finding.

After that, specifically comment on:

- absence of stigmata of CLD, as this is the most common cause for hepatomegaly
- signs of right-sided heart failure, especially peripheral oedema and raised jugular venous pressure (JVP)
- signs that could accompany a possible malignant or inflammatory process, such as cachexia and lymphadenopathy; and
- absence of other organomegaly, such as splenomegaly.

MNEMONIC

Hepatomegaly – causes: $C_3I_2A_2$

Cirrhosis (CLD)

Congestive cardiac failure

Cancer (liver, metastatic, haematological)

Infection (hepatitis, hydatid cyst, amoebic/pyogenic abscess

Infiltration (sarcoidosis, amyloidosis, storage diseases)

Artery (vascular disease or blood disease)

Alcoholic hepatitis

Workup

- Full history, including constitutional symptoms, travel, cardiac and social histories
- Routine blood investigations
- Liver screen
- Infection screen
- Abdominal ultrasound with Doppler studies of the hepatic and portal veins.

Model presentation

This patient, who presents with abdominal discomfort, has hepatomegaly on clinical examination. His liver edge is palpable 6 cm below the costal margin, which is nontender, hard and regular on palpation. There are no bruits over the palpable liver.

There is no other obvious organomegaly on examination, and specifically no splenomegaly.

There are no peripheral stigmata of CLD.

There is no obvious lymphadenopathy; however, I have not formally assessed for inguinal, axillary or cervical lymph nodes.

There are no signs of heart failure or sepsis.

In summary, this patient has hepatomegaly, but the absence of other signs on clinical examination has not enabled me to identify an underlying aetiology for this. The differential list includes CLD, cardiac failure, malignancy, viral and parasitic infections, storage diseases and vascular liver diseases.

I would like to finish my assessment by looking at the observation chart and temperature record, and taking further history, including other symptoms, cardiac, travel, family and social histories.

Initially I would request some blood tests and request a liver ultrasound with Doppler studies.

Discussion with the examiners

If you get this case, the discussion with the examiners will probably be shaped along the lines of CLD (see relevant case).

> **Tip!**
>
> This should be an easy case; the only action you definitely need to take is to identify the hepatomegaly. It is very important to practise identifying organomegaly, as in the absence of stigmata of CLD, you may lose a case like this. The technique should be practised well, as the examiners will not forgive missing this sign.
>
> *Percussion*: Should be performed in the midclavicular line. Use heavy percussion to identify the upper border, and light percussion for the lower edge.
>
> *Palpation*: Should be performed with your hand in the midclavicular line and parallel to the transverse rectus abdominis muscle, starting below the liver edge, and moving up with each exhaled breath until the liver edge meets your fingers.
>
> During palpation, you should be positioned at the same level as the patient's abdomen.

Splenomegaly

Presenting a case of *splenomegaly without hepatomegaly*

Positive clinical findings

When you present a patient with lone splenomegaly, do not present findings in the order in which you did or did not elicit them, as you may lose time presenting many negative findings. This could bore the examiners, and may lead to marks unnecessarily being lost. Instead, start your presentation with the splenomegaly finding itself: 'This patient, who presented with abdominal pain, has splenomegaly/enlarged spleen on abdominal palpation, with the splenic tip lying 5 cm below the costal margin.'

MNEMONIC

Causes of lone splenomegaly: *HARP*

*H*aematological malignancies
*A*naemia – haemolytic
*R*heumatoid arthritis (Felty)
*P*ortal hypertension

Presence of signs revealing the underlying diagnosis (important positive and important negative signs):

After presenting splenomegaly as your finding, go on with your presentation, referring to the presence or absence of important signs that may reveal the underlying cause of this patient's splenomegaly.

- Haematological malignancy:
  - Anaemia
  - Lymphadenopathy
  - Cachexia.
- Portal hypertension:
  - Evidence of CLD.
- Felty's syndrome:
  - Evidence of rheumatological disease.
- Haemolytic anaemia:
  - Jaundice.

The differential diagnosis for lone splenomegaly is large, including:

- Infections:
  - Brucella, salmonella, leishmania
  - Endocarditis
  - Tuberculosis
  - Epstein–Barr virus.
- Storage diseases:
  - Amyloidosis
  - Sarcoidosis.
- Autoimmune diseases:
  - Systematic lupus erythematous.

but these causes rarely appear in the exam.

Workup

- Detailed history including travel and sexual histories, as well as presence of constitutional symptoms (weight loss, fevers, sweats)
- Blood investigations
- Abdominal USS
- Axial imaging.

Model presentation

This patient presents with abdominal pain, and on examination there is splenomegaly without hepatomegaly. There is no evidence of anaemia or jaundice, reducing the possibility of a myeloproliferative disorder or haemolytic anaemia. There are no stigmata of CLD or portal hypertension. There are no signs of rheumatoid arthritis, or signs of any connective tissue disorder, but there is lymphadenopathy, possibly representing an underlying lymphoproliferative disorder, such as chronic lymphocytic leukaemia (CLL).

I would like to conclude my examination by examining for inguinal, axillary and cervical lymphadenopathy, and take a detailed history, including travel history and constitutional symptoms, as well as symptoms of cytopaenia, infections, bleeding, anaemia, autoimmune or liver disease. I would like to request an USS of the abdomen to confirm my finding of splenomegaly, and run some initial blood tests.

Discussion with the examiners

How would you proceed investigating this patient?
- Blood tests:
  - FBC and blood film
  - Serum LDH
  - β2 Microglobulin
  - Autoimmune profile
  - HIV testing.
- Imaging:
  - Start with an abdominal USS to confirm your diagnosis of splenomegaly, and at the same time visualize the liver and the portal system
  - Axial imaging.
- Other investigations:
  - Lymph node biopsy
  - Bone marrow biopsy.

How would you manage this patient?
In the first instance, you would treat the confirmed diagnosis and refer to the relevant specialty. Below are management strategies for some of the conditions that can cause lone splenomegaly, but examiners will not expect you to know any of these treatments in detail.

Haematological malignancy

Cases appearing at this station are myeloproliferative disorders, most commonly CML, and lymphoproliferative disorders, most commonly CLL.

- Chronic lymphocytic leukaemia:
  - caused by monoclonal proliferation of well differentiated B lymphocytes
  - blood film shows smudge cells, and immunophenotyping reveals CD19, CD20
  - recognized complications:
    - hypogammaglobulinaemia
    - warm autoimmune haemolytic anaemia
    - transformation to high-grade lymphoma.
  - indications for treating a patient with chemotherapy:
    - progressive marrow failure or progressive lymphocytosis
    - massive lymphadenopathy or massive splenomegaly
    - systemic symptoms
    - autoimmune cytopaenias.
- Chronic myeloid leukaemia (CML):
  - Philadelphia chromosome: t(9;22)(q34;q11)
  - Ph chromosome is identified by PCR; blood and bone marrow examinations reveal lots of cells with all grades of maturation
  - Patients exhibit three clinical stages of disease:
    - Benign chronic stage:
      - asymptomatic or nonspecific symptoms.
    - Accelerated stage:
      - unwell
      - weight loss
      - organomegaly.
    - Late stage:
      - blastic crisis with transformation to acute leukaemia.

Haemolytic anaemia

Anaemia is caused by a reduced lifetime of red blood cells. They can be acute or chronic. The cause of haemolysis can be congenital or acquired. Haemolysis (destruction of red blood cells) can happen intravascularly, as in some autoimmune haemolytic anaemias, certain red cell syndromes, in G6PD deficiency with stress and in transfusion reactions.

> **Tip!**
> Patients with chronic haemolytic anaemia often have gallstones, so a cholecystectomy scar can be a clue to the underlying diagnosis.

When would you consider splenectomy for a patient?

Splenectomy is a high-risk operation, and it is rarely curative for a medical disease, so is only considered under specific circumstances. Diseases that may have an indication for splenectomy (apart from splenic rupture) are in general severe haematological genetic conditions that have haemolysis/hypersplenism as one of their features (idiopathic thrombocytopenic purpura [ITP], sickle-cell disease, haemolytic anaemia and hereditary spherocytosis).

Renal

Renal transplant

Presenting a case of a *renal transplant*

Organize your presentation into two parts:

Part 1. Describe the presence of the renal graft

Start your presentation describing the finding of the transplant itself, describing the scar you noted on your inspection, and the mass you felt on palpation, as well as the presence or absence of any bruits on auscultation above the mass.

Part 2. Present important positive and negative findings

> **Tip!**
> When you have identified a renal transplant, to impress the examiners and get full marks, you should comment on five things:
> 1. Is the graft working?
> 2. Evidence of previous renal replacement therapy (RRT) modes.
> 3. Signs of immunosuppression.
> 4. Complications of patient's renal disease.
> 5. Identifiable possible cause for the patient's renal disease.

The way to answer to all these questions is within your presentation.
- Is the graft working?
  - The graft is (or is not) working because there are (no) signs of uraemia, the patient is euvolaemic (oedematous), and there are (no) other current alternative methods of RRT.
- What are the previous RRT modes?
  - Scars on the chest from previous sites of vascular access
  - Unused or nonfunctioning fistulas on the arms
  - Abdominal scars from previous peritoneal dialysis.
- Are there signs of immunosuppression?
  - Gum hypertrophy
  - Cushingoid signs
  - Skin warts (papillomas)
  - Hand tremors.

- Are there any complications of the end-stage renal failure (ESRF)?
  - Signs of anaemia
  - Signs of hyperparathyroidism
  - Scars from parathyroidectomy.
- Possible causes of ESRF:
  - Diabetes mellitus (look for evidence of pinpricks on patient's fingertips)
  - Hypertension
  - Polycystic kidney disease (palpable polycystic kidneys or nephrectomy scars)
  - Systemic lupus erythematosus (SLE) (signs of SLE).

Model presentation

This patient has a scar in his right iliac fossa. Below the scar, there is a smooth, firm, nontender palpable mass. There are no bruits on auscultation.

This patient has a renal transplant, a treatment for ESRF. The transplant appears to be functioning well as the patient has no signs of uraemia or fluid overload on examination, and there are currently no other functioning modalities of RRT.

Prior to the transplant the patient was on haemodialysis, as evident by a nonfunctioning fistula (or a functioning fistula with no signs of recent needling in his left arm).

The patient is on steroids, as is evident by Cushingoid features.

His renal failure may have been complicated with tertiary hyperparathyroidism, as there appears to be a surgery scar on his neck.

I would like to complete my examination by measuring the patient's blood pressure and perform a dipstick analysis of his urine. I would like to obtain a detailed history of the patient's symptoms, including past medical history, and then I would proceed with investigations, specifically blood tests for renal function and electrolytes, an ultrasound scan of the transplanted kidney, and immunosuppressant levels.

Discussion with the examiners

What investigations would you request for this patient?

The most probable candidate information for this patient would be, 'This patient presents with abdominal pain. Please examine his/her abdomen.'

After identifying the presence of a kidney transplant, your investigations should initially be concerned with the function of the transplant.

- Blood tests:
  - Full blood count (FBC), biochemical profile, clotting and inflammatory markers
  - Immunosuppressant levels.
- Urinalysis:
  - Test for blood, protein or infection.
- Imaging:
  - Ultrasound +/− Doppler.
- Consider a biopsy if indicated.

There is a long list of investigations that may follow these initial tests, but for the purposes of this exam, the examiners will not expect more detail.

What are the complications of renal transplant?

1. Infection:
   - More prone to usual bacterial infections.
   - Cytomegalovirus, Pneumocystis pneumonia.
2. Malignancies:
   - Post-transplant lympho-proliferative disease.
   - Skin-cancer-like squamous cell carcinoma.

Name some common immunosuppressant medications in renal transplant

- Prednisolone
- Tacrolimus
- Sirolimus
- Cyclosporin
- Mycophenolate.

How would you manage this patient?

For the management of a case like this, the examiners might pose a wide range of questions related to renal failure.

The most common questions are:

- General management principles in chronic renal disease.
- For chronic kidney disease (CKD), patients should be monitored closely in renal clinics, and treatment is directed toward

- managing the underlying cause:
  - controlling hypertension; and
  - managing diabetes.
- Slowing the disease progression with medications with prognostic benefit (ACE-inhibitors).
- Managing cardiovascular risk factors (smoking cessation, aspirin, statins).
- Managing the electrolyte and metabolic complications of CKD, and
  - vitamin D deficiency
  - metabolic acidosis
  - hyperkalaemia
  - hyperphosphataemia; and
  - volume overload.
- Managing anaemia with iron or erythropoietin.
- In acute kidney injury, the immediate management is to:
  - Stop nephrotoxic medications
  - Assess urine output
  - Manage fluid balance; and
  - Establish the cause of renal failure:
    - pre-renal: assess fluid status and obtain detailed history
    - renal: diagnose with blood tests and renal biopsy; and
    - post-renal: obtain imaging (USS, CT).

Urgent haemodialysis has a place in the management of acute renal failure, if complications are present:
- hyperkalaemia
- volume overload/pulmonary odaema
- clinical uraema, pericarditis, encephalopathy
- severe acidosis.

Adult polycystic kidney disease

Presenting a case of APKD

If your diagnosis is adult polycystic kidney disease (APKD), begin your presentation with your main abdominal finding of the polycystic kidneys. 'There are bilateral flank masses. The masses are ballotable; you can get above them, and the overlying percussion note is resonant.'

Tip!

After presenting the diagnosis of APKD, you have to comment on the next four things:

1. Are there any replacement modes of renal function? (see 'Renal transplant' section)
2. Is there any other evident organomegaly? (liver/spleen)
3. Are there any complications of CKD?
   Uraemia, hypervolaemia, anaemia
4. Comment on possible nephrectomy scars.

This will give the examiners the confidence that you have really looked for all the relevant findings, which means you really know what to expect when reviewing a patient with such a diagnosis.

Then complete your presentation by saying that you would like to look at other features associated with APKD, and for that reason you would like to measure the patient's blood pressure, and examine the patient's cardiovascular and neurological systems.

MNEMONIC

Possible complications of APKD: CA_3MP

Cysts in other organs (liver)

Anaemia

Abdominal pain (if a cyst bleeds or gets infected)

Aneurysms in brain

Mitral valve prolapse

Polycythaemia

Workup

- KUB ultrasound
- Biochemical profile (BCP)
- FBC
- Urine dip
- CT to look for infection or haemorrhage.

Model presentation

This patient, who presented with abdominal pain, has bilateral flank masses on examination of her abdomen. These masses are ballotable. The percussion note above both masses is resonant. In summary, this patient's clinical examination is consistent with adult polycystic kidney disease (APKD). The patient does not have any evidence of RRT, as there are no arteriovenous fistulas in her arms, there are no tunnelled catheters in situ, and no signs of either current peritoneal dialysis or transplanted kidney. I could not appreciate any evidence of hepatomegaly consistent with hepatic cysts. She appears to be euvolaemic, and there is no uraemic flap on outstretched hands. There is no evidence of anaemia.

I would like to complete my examination by looking at the observation chart, check the blood pressure, perform a urine dip and a complete cardiovascular and neurological examination to search for extra-renal complications of her condition.

The pain she presented with today may be due to intra-cyst haemorrhage or infection, and I would like to investigate further for that.

Discussion with the examiners

What are other possible differentials for bilateral palpable kidneys?

1. Bilateral hydronephrosis
2. Amyloidosis
3. Renal cell carcinoma
4. Bilateral kidney cysts
   Tuberous sclerosis
   Von Hippel Lindau.

How is APKD inherited?

- Autosomal dominant condition:
  - ADPKD1 in chromosome 16
  - ADPKD2 in chromosome 4
  - Rarely spontaneous mutation.
- Autosomal recessive is almost nonexisting in APKD.

What are the ultrasound diagnostic criteria in people with positive family history of ADPKD?

- <30 years old: at least two unilateral or bilateral cysts (consider rescanning after 30 years old if criteria not met)

- 30–60 years old: two cysts in each kidney
- >60 years old: more than four cysts in each kidney.

Genetic testing is rarely used for diagnosis.

What is the management of ADPKD?

- No treatment has been proven to slow the progression of the disease to date.
- Treat hypertension and hyperlipidaemia.
- Promptly manage infections and abdominal pain episodes.
- Refer to renal team for followup and consideration of RRT if applicable.
- Counselling, offer screening to family members.
- Screen for intracerebral aneurysm (ICA) if there is family history of ICA or previous ruptured ICA.

Where to find renal cases for practise

The best place is the renal ward, the renal clinics and the dialysis unit in your hospital.

History taking

Station 2 assesses history-taking skills and, apart from rare exceptions, will be one of four different categories of case:

1. A specific new symptom (e.g. dyspnea)
2. A known chronic disease followup (e.g. rheumatoid arthritis)
3. A combination of symptoms (e.g. weight loss and tiredness)
4. An incidental investigation finding (e.g. high calcium).

We will present example cases from each of these categories, as well as a detailed strategy on how to utilize your time efficiently during the station to achieve maximum marks. The structure of the example cases can be applied to any case that may come up in Station 2.

Station 2, as well as being relatively easy to pass, is a great opportunity for candidates to achieve full marks, which can be useful in compensating for the other, more difficult, stations.

This is especially true if you put in lots of pre-exam practice. Candidates who have prepared well come across as fluent and confident in the actual exam and score well.

Station 2 begins before you actually see a patient. As soon as Station 1 finishes and the bell rings, take full advantage of the 5 minutes given before you enter the room. Read the case carefully and thoroughly and try to decide:

1. Into which of the categories does this case fit?
2. If it is a new symptom or a combination of symptoms, what are the possible differential diagnoses?
3. What questions should I ask to help me confirm or rule out my list of differential diagnoses/complications?
4. How am I going to best summarize my consultation to appear as smooth as possible?

Use the preparation time to jot down notes on these questions, as this will help in creating the skeleton of your consultation.

When you enter the station, introduce yourself to the patient/surrogate and then start with an open question. A good way is to repeat the information provided to you, making sure it is correct, and ask the patient to tell you more about it. This way, the patient will be able to volunteer much of the information they are allowed to, which will guide your subsequent direct questioning. Having a list of differentials in your head from the preparation time will allow you to then ask closed questions that will confirm or rule out a diagnosis/complication.

> **Tip!**
> Starting with an open question and then asking more focused, direct questions mirrors the natural flow of a good consultation and appears slick to the examiners.

Continue the consultation with more closed questions to the patient, targeted toward possible diagnosis, with exclusion of possible differentials, and follow the skeleton that you have created in your notes before entering the station, but make sure the consultation has a natural flow as well.

Always allow the patient/surrogate some time to express their concerns regarding the underlying presenting complaint, and if they have not done so by themselves, do ask them directly about their concerns. You cannot assume what their worries are, as their agenda may not match yours. Failing to address the patient's concerns will result in you scoring 'unsatisfactory' in some of the station's domains.

When you are warned by the examiners that you have 2 minutes left, start explaining to the patient what your diagnosis is, what the other possible differentials are (if any), and what the management plan is for the patient from now on (hospital admission/investigations/re-review in clinic/refer to another specialty, etc.).

The examiners are marking you for the rapport you have with your patient, and the patient leaving the room having fully understood what the management plan is, is part of this rapport.

Finishing your summary, do ask the patient once again if they have anything else to mention that has not been already covered, if there is something they have not entirely understood, or if they have any other concerns that have not been addressed so far. If you have time, do address them, but if you have run out of time, make sure you explain to the patient that you will see them again, after some investigations have taken place, and you will be addressing anything left in the next consultation.

The clinical domains that you are marked on during this station are:
- clinical communication skills
- managing patient's concerns
- differential diagnosis
- clinical judgment; and
- maintaining patient's welfare.

An important thing to have in mind is that the first two domains are not tested in all stations, but only in Stations 2, 4 and 5. For each of these domains you can score a maximum of 16 points, with 10 points being the minimum score required to pass. One-third of the points in these domains come from Station 2. Given that, the opportunity to score 'satisfactory' in these domains is given to you only four of the eight total times you will be examined, you must be very careful, aiming to achieve full marks by both examiners in both domains during Station 2, which is the easiest amongst Stations 2, 4 and 5. The way to achieve full marks in both domains is to practise your consultation skills in different scenarios, making sure you follow a routine that is sleek, and give the surrogate the opportunity to express their concerns in a manner that does not disrupt the flow of the consultation itself. Also remember that giving the opportunity to the patient to address their concerns is not enough to give you satisfactory marks. The examiners have to actively see you attempting to address and manage those concerns in any way you can within the limitations of a 14-minute consultation. If the patient has a question that cannot be answered because of lack of information at the time, just be honest with the patient, telling him or her that you would like to revisit this matter when more investigations are available, or when you have a definite diagnosis for them. Do not attempt to give false information or false hope to the patient.

The next cases are examples of each category that can appear in the PACES exam. Each has a suggested strategy on how to utilize your time during the station to achieve full marks. If you find these models useful, you can apply them to any case that may come up in the history station.

Once you have finished your summary, ask the patient if there is anything you haven't covered or if he or she has any other questions. There are always marks for asking how the symptoms have affected the patient (work, family) so always ask what effect these symptoms have had on the patient's daily life.

After 14 minutes, the patient/surrogate will leave the room and you will get 1 minute to gather your thoughts and prepare for the examiners questions. The examiners will have 5 minutes to ask you any questions on the case, and these are usually:

- present the case
- present the patient's problem list
- present your differential diagnosis; and
- present you management plan, including investigations and treatment.

The questions will be strictly related to the domains on which the examiners are asked to mark you, and will consist of your diagnosis and the patient's concerns, the investigations and the treatment you have to propose.

Single presenting complaint: Shortness of breath

Referral letter
Dear Doctor,
Thank you for seeing this patient, who presented to our practice with a history of worsening shortness of breath over the last month.
I would appreciate your opinion regarding diagnosis and further management.
Kind Regards,
Dr Kelly (GP)

Preparation before entering the examination room

Before entering the room, take the advantage of the 5 minutes given to prepare, and make two sets of notes on a piece of paper. On one side, write all possible differentials you have in mind after reading the letter: for example, 'interstitial lung disease, chronic obstructive pulmonary disease, cardiac failure, asthma, pulmonary embolism, functional'.

On the other side, write down the skeleton of your consultation, which will consist of the traditional model of: 'presenting complaint, history of presenting complaint, past medical history, drug history including allergies, social history, family history and specific enquiry/system review'. On this side, always include 'patient's questions/concerns'.

In the examination room

Presenting complaint

Once you have entered the room and have introduced yourself to the examiners and the patient, start the history taking with an open question toward the patient. Repeat the presenting complaint that you know from reading the referral letter, and ask the patient to tell you more about it. In this answer, the patient will be volunteering all the information they are allowed to before your direct questioning. This will guide you toward a differential list already.

After you have confirmed understanding that the patient's presenting complaint matches the information you have been given in the referral letter, continue with closed questions, regarding details about the specific symptom, characteristics, progression and status of the disease, as well as the presence of other associated symptoms that have not already been volunteered.

History of presenting complaint/associated symptoms

- When did the shortness of breath start?
- When was the last time you were well?
- Has the shortness of breath become gradually worse during this period of time?
- Before noticing the shortness of breath, how far could you walk without stopping?
- How far can you walk now before getting out of breath?
- Pattern of dyspnea? Do you feel more out of breath some times of the day than others (when at work? in bed? more in the afternoon?)?
- Paroxysmal nocturnal dyspnea? Orthopnoea?
- Precipitating factors? Have you noticed any specific activities or factors that make your breathing worse or better?

Ask for any (relevant to the main presenting complaint) associated symptoms, like:
- chest pains
- palpitations
- ankle oedema
- wheeze
- cough (dry/productive)
- sputum
- fevers
- weight loss; and
- night sweats.

> **Tip!**
>
> Asking about associated symptoms that are relevant to the main presenting complaint should come after the initial questioning about the main symptom. Any other symptoms that are not relevant initially, or are not immediately related to your initial differential diagnosis list, are best left for the very end of the consultation, when you reach the systemic enquiry phase.

Past medical history/family history/drug history/social history

Depending on the character of the symptom and the differential diagnosis that you have in mind, you have to concentrate on specific aspects of the patient's symptomatology prior to the initial presentation. For instance, for the dyspnea case, you have to take a detailed respiratory history of:

- asbestos or other dust exposure
- smoking history
- travel history
- pets at home
- occupation
- past medical history of lung or heart disease
- risk factors for pulmonary embolism
- contact with known tuberculosis; and
- medication list and allergies.

By this time, you should have a clear idea of the most likely diagnosis, as well as the top two to three differentials. Here is the time to ask any other questions that will help you formulate the ultimate working diagnosis. If you need more details of a specific symptom that you have discovered, here is the time to ask for it.

Make sure you ask the patient whether they want to report any other symptoms that you have not asked of.

> **Tip!**
>
> During this station, the examiners are marking you in five different domains: communication, clinical judgment, differential diagnosis, managing patient's concerns and maintaining patient's welfare.
>
> So far, during your consultation, you will have had the opportunity to score only on the first domain. The rest of the domains will be scored within a shorter amount of time, so it is crucial to make sure you cover them after the first half of your consultation.

> **Tip!**
>
> *Explore patient's concerns*: The patient will have two to three direct questions in their agenda to ask you. Give them the opportunity to ask, so that when you summarize your thoughts to the patient, you make sure you address these questions as well. You should not forget to mention these concerns when you present the case to the examiners. The concerns should definitely form part of the patient's problem list. Do not assume you know what the patient's concerns are, as the examiners have to listen to you asking the direct question. The patient's concerns may be totally different than the ones you assume, so make sure you ask the question and then address their concerns.

When you are warned by the examiners that you have 2 minutes left, start explaining to the patient what your working diagnosis is, what the possible differentials are, if any, and what the management plan is for the patient from now on (admission, investigations and re-review in clinic, refer to another specialty, etc.). During this period of time, you have the opportunity to be marked on the domains of clinical judgment and differential diagnosis.

Finishing your summary, ask the patient once again if they have anything else to report that you have not covered or if they have any other questions.

Chronic condition: Known rheumatoid arthritis, uncontrolled symptoms

---

Referral letter

Dear Doctor,

Thank you for seeing this patient, who has been diagnosed with rheumatoid arthritis some years ago.

She is currently on regular analgesia, which fails to control her symptoms. She came today asking if we can give her a course of steroids, as this has helped her in the past.

I would appreciate your opinion on further management.

Kind Regards,

Dr Kelly (GP)

Before entering the examination room

Chronic diseases are best managed in this station in two parts. Write down questions for these two parts on the piece of paper provided.

The first part consists of details of the acute presentation, specifically establishing whether this presentation is part of the chronic disease the patient has been diagnosed with.

The second part consists of details of the course of the disease from onset until this consultation. Although this type of case seems to be a difficult one, in reality, it is the simplest type of case that can come up in this station, as the patient or surrogate will be able to provide details of the disease progression so far.

In the examination room

Presenting complaint/history of presenting complaint

Always start with an open question first. Repeat the presenting complaint that you know, and ask the patient to tell you more about it. In this answer, the patient will be volunteering all the information they are allowed to before your direct questioning, and this will guide you toward a differential list.

After the initial open question, proceed to closed questioning, including specifics of progression of the disease between the last clinic visit and today, including musculoskeletal and more systemic symptoms.

- Which joints are involved?
- What is the pattern of the pain?
- Do you still get stiffness in the mornings?
- Which tasks could you perform prior to the previous clinic? Which tasks are restricted now?
- What is the progression pattern through this time? Gradually getting worse? Or alternating good and bad days?
- Have you had any problems with your eyes, like red or dry eyes?
- Have you felt more out of breath than usual during this period of time?
- Have you been getting any pins and needles feeling across your legs or arms?
- Have you had any rashes on your skin that you've noticed?

Past medical history/progression of the disease from diagnosis to present

Flashback: ask the patient to give you a detailed timeline of deteriorations, events and medications since their diagnosis, and try to identify any pattern of worsening (medications stopped or tapered down, acute illness exacerbating the existing disease, intolerance to specific medications, noncompliance).

- When were you diagnosed with rheumatoid arthritis?
- Who has looked after your arthritis since?
- How often have you had flare-ups of your condition?
- How did you manage these flare-ups?
- What medications have you used in the past?
- When was the last time you saw a consultant in clinic? What did they tell you?
- Have you been taking your medications since?

> **Tip!**
> When the scenario involves a patient with a known disease that presents with uncontrolled symptoms, noncompliance with currently prescribed medications can be a common differential that you have to explore in detail during the consultation.

Go into detailed history about current medications and try to identify any compliance issues due to medication side effects.

- Which medications are you taking at the moment?
- Have you had any side effects from any of these medications?
- Have any of the medications you are currently taking made you feel nauseated? (The most common side effects that patients on disease-modifying anti-rheumatic drugs experience is nausea.)

Other past medical history/social history/family history

Do not forget to go through a systemic enquiry of all organ systems asking about systemic symptoms that can occur with rheumatic disease and ask about other past medical history.

Patient's concerns

Concentrate on interference of their disease with quality of life and ask the patient what their concerns are.

When you are warned by the examiners that you have 2 minutes left, start explaining to the patient what your diagnosis is, what the possible differentials are, if any, and what the management plan is for the patient from now on (admission, investigations and re-review in clinic, refer to another specialty, etc.).

Finishing your summary, ask the patient once again if they have anything else to report that you have not covered, or if they have any other questions.

At the end of the 14 minutes, the patient/surrogate will leave the room, you will get 1 minute to gather your findings/thoughts, and then you will be answering examiners' questions on the case.

Mixture of different symptoms: Weight loss and tiredness

Referral letter
Dear Doctor,
Thank you for seeing this patient, who presented with a combination of weight loss and tiredness for the last year.
His BMI today was 17.5, which is in the range of 'underweight'.
I would appreciate your opinion regarding diagnosis and further management.
Kind Regards,
Dr Kelly (GP)

Preparation before entering the examination room

Before entering the examination room, try to create a list of differential diagnoses that can account for the combination of these symptoms. For each differential, generate a list of symptoms to ask for once you enter the room. The patient will have received specific instructions to give answers on the presence or absence of symptoms only if asked.

As before, making a list using the traditional model of history taking will help you appear systematic and fluent within the clinical consultation.

In the examination room

Presenting complaint

Always start with an open question first. Repeat the presenting complaint that you know, and ask the patient to tell you more about it. In this answer, the patient will be volunteering all the information they are allowed to before your direct questioning, and this will guide you toward a differential list already. Remember to ask about each complaint mentioned in the letter separately, and try to figure out the timeline in terms of which symptom appeared first, as a different order of symptom appearance will sometimes guide you toward a different diagnosis.

History of presenting complaint

Quantify the weight loss, and ask specifically the time period over which the weight loss has occurred.

- How much weight would you say you have lost?
- Have you weighed yourself recently? How many clothing sizes have you dropped?
- Since when have you noticed that you have been losing weight?
- Over this period of time, how many kilograms have you lost?
- How about the tiredness? How long have you been feeling more tired than usual?
- Have you been feeling tired throughout the day or do you find that you wake up tired and you feel re-energized as the day progresses?
- Has this tiredness made you take days off work? How many and how often?
- Have you felt more sleepy during the day? Have you fallen asleep during the day while doing activities where you are not supposed to sleep?
- What has the quality of your sleep been like? What is it that makes you wake up at night?
- Have you had to abandon activities that you used to do because of these symptoms?

Associated symptoms

- Is the weight loss fully unintentional?
- How has your appetite been throughout this time?
- How are your bowel habits? Have you noticed any change in your bowel habits? If the answer is positive, ask specifically about constipation or diarrhoea, with details about appearance and frequency.
- Have you noticed if you are losing blood from anywhere? Any blood in your bowel motions, or when you pass water? Have you coughed up any blood? Have you ever vomited blood?
- Have you had any nausea/vomiting?
- Have you had any problems swallowing food? Does it feel as if the food is stuck in your gullet, or is it painful when you swallow? Is this feeling

only with solid foods or equally bad both with solid foods and liquids, like water?

- Have you had any fevers that you've noticed? If so, ask for specific patterns of fever.
- Do you get any night sweats? Have you ever woken up at night drenched in sweat? How often?
- Have you noticed any lumps or bumps in your body?
- Have you been experiencing any pains anywhere? Chest pains? Abdominal pains? Muscle aches? Bone pains? Back pain? Joint pains?
- Have you had any palpitations?
- Have you noticed your appetite has increased despite losing weight?
- Have you noticed that you cannot tolerate hot environments as well as you did before?
- Have you noticed any changes in your skin?
- Have you had any back pain recently?
- Have you been out of breath more than usual? Have you been coughing up anything?

Once you have covered all the information you need to help in creating a list of two or three differentials, then you can go on with the traditional model.

Past medical/family/social history/drug history and allergies

Ask about detailed occupational history, travel history and social history, including smoking and alcohol, and enquire specifically about infections and haematological diseases.

Explore the patient's concerns

When you are warned by the examiners that you have 2 minutes left, start explaining to the patient what your diagnosis is, what the possible differentials are, if any, and what the management plan is for the patient from now on (admission, investigations and re-review in clinic, refer to another specialty, etc.).

Finishing your summary, ask the patient once again if they have anything else to report that you have not covered, or if they have any other questions.

At the end of the 14 minutes, the patient/surrogate will leave the room, you will get 1 minute to gather your findings/thoughts, and then you will be answering examiners' questions on the case.

Investigation finding: Hypercalcaemia

Referral letter
Dear Doctor,
Thank you for seeing this patient, who was found to have high calcium levels on recent routine blood tests.
I would appreciate your opinion regarding further investigations and management.
Kind Regards,
Dr Kelly (GP)

Preparation before entering the examination room

Before entering the examination room, write down a list of the possible differentials for hypercalcaemia, and a separate list of symptoms that hypercalcaemia can give rise to. Prepare yourself to ask two sets of questions at the start of the consultation: one set of questions involving details of hypercalcaemia-specific symptoms, and one set involving details of cause-specific symptoms and information.

In the examination room

Before mentioning the finding to the patient, ask more detail about the background of why the investigation was undertaken. Although in the exam setting the patient/surrogate will know about the specific result, as they have been briefed on the case, in the real setting the patient may not really know or understand what the abnormal result means. Because you are assessed on your communication skills at the same time in this station, it is best for the examiners to see that you know how to start similar consultations in real life.

So, instead of repeating the information you are given as with all other three types of cases, it is best to establish what the patient knows first. Start with a generic statement such as:

'Your doctor has written to me informing me that you recently had some blood tests. Can you tell me why these blood tests were organized?'

In this case, the patient will answer that they have had routine blood tests; however, in cases of 'abnormal result referral', the abnormal finding may be either an incidental finding that warrants further attention or an investigation that was specifically requested after a patient complained of a specific symptom, in which case you need to establish that both you and the patient know why the test was taken in the first place, as well as understanding of the result of the investigation. At that point, for this scenario, you can explain to the patient what the abnormal finding was:

'These tests showed the calcium level in your blood is high. The reason you are here is for us to try to find out why and whether we need to look further into this.'

History of presenting complaint

After this introduction, ask the patient about symptoms related to the finding and possible underlying causes that could have given rise to this finding.

- When was the last time before this occasion that you had blood tests taken? Was everything normal back then?
- Have you had any tummy pains during the last months? Do these pains ever go into your back or your sides? How often have you had them? Have you seen a doctor about these pains? Have you taken anything for the pain?
- Have you ever noticed any blood in your urine?
- Have you had any pains in your muscles or deep within your bones? When was the first time you noticed those pains? Do they come and go, or are they always there? Have those pains ever woken you up from sleep?
- Have you noticed lately that you have been feeling more thirsty than usual? How much water would you say you are drinking daily? Was this the case 6 months ago?
- Have you or your friends and relatives noticed any change in your behaviour recently?
- Have you noticed any lumps in your neck?
- Have you had any chest pain or palpitations in the last months? How often? Have you felt dizzy or blacked out with these palpitations?
- Have you lost weight recently? If so, how much and over what period of time?
- Have you been feeling more out of breath than normal? Have you been coughing anything up? Any blood that you have noticed in your sputum?

- Have you noticed any changes in your bowel habits?
- Have you had any problems with your urinary output?

Past medical history/family history/social history
- Have you ever had any problem with your blood?
- Have you ever had high calcium levels before?
- Have you ever been diagnosed with cancer?
- Are there any other members in your family that have been told that they have high calcium levels?
- Do you smoke? How many cigarettes per day? For how many years have you been a smoker?
- How much alcohol do you normally drink?

Drug history and allergies
Very often, when a blood test comes back as abnormal, it may represent nothing more than an adverse effect of a medication. It is essential that you take a detailed drug history from the patient, including both prescribed medications and other medication use. Ask questions like:
- What medications do you take regularly?
- Do you take any prescribed, or over-the-counter, medications for your stomach?
- Do you take any dietary supplements, like vitamins or minerals? Are you on calcium tablets?

Patient's concerns
Explore the patient's concerns with direct questioning:
- Is there anything that particularly worries/concerns you at this point?
- Do you have any questions for me?

Explain the plan
When you are warned by the examiners that you have 2 minutes left, start explaining to the patient what your working diagnosis is, what the possible differentials are, if any, and what the management plan is for the patient from now on (admission, investigations and re-review in clinic, refer to another specialty, etc.). During this period of time, you have the opportunity to be assessed in the domains of 'clinical judgment' and 'differential diagnosis'.

   Finishing your summary, ask the patient once again if they have anything else to report that you have not covered, or if they have any other questions.

At the end of the 14 minutes, the patient/surrogate will leave the room, you will get 1 minute to gather your findings/thoughts, and then you will be answering examiners' questions on the case.

Exercise 1

Information for the candidate

Patient details: Miss Apple, 21 years old

Your role: You are the core medical trainee year 2 (CMT2) doctor in the general medical outpatient clinic.

Please read the referral letter from the patient's GP. You will have 5 minutes to read the letter and take any notes, 14 minutes to take the history from the patient, 1 minute to collect your thoughts and 5 minutes with the examiners. You may take the notes with you in the examination room.

Referral letter

Dear Doctor,

Thank you for seeing this lady, who presented with a history of witnessed collapse episodes over the last month.

She is otherwise fit and well, and has no other past medical history of note.

I would appreciate your opinion regarding the cause of her collapses, and your advice on further management.

Kind Regards,

Dr Kelly

Information for the patient

You are Miss Penny Apple, 21 years old.

Over the last 4 weeks, you have collapsed on three occasions. The first time was whilst on holiday in Crete. You were playing on the beach with your friends and the next thing you remember is lying on the sand and people around you asking if you were okay. You refused to go to the hospital at the time because you were not feeling unwell. You thought it must have been the hot weather that caused the blackout.

The second time also happened in Crete while you were hiking in the mountains. The weather was also very hot that day. You refused to go and get medical attention as you did not want to ruin anyone else's holiday.

The last time happened last week while back in the United Kingdom and helping one of your friends in the garden. They convinced you to go to the doctor.

Prior to these episodes you do not feel light-headed and you get no warning of an impending faint. You do not get chest pain, shortness of breath or palpitations. You never get a headache.

Your friend told you that you were unconscious for a few seconds and no one has mentioned seeing any jerking movements or fitting.

You have never injured yourself, bitten your tongue or been incontinent.

When you come around, you can tell who you are, what you were doing before collapsing and where you are, but on no occasion do you remember actually falling.

You are on no regular medications and have no allergies.

You do not smoke and only drink alcohol occasionally. You have never used illicit drugs. You do not have a driving licence. You have no illnesses that you are aware of and have never had to go to hospital before.

You are an only child and both parents are fit and well. You lost an uncle on your mother's side when he was in his 20s. You had heard that there was a problem with his heart but don't know any further details.

Your questions to the doctor

You want to know whether you have epilepsy, as one of your friends had something similar and she was told she has epilepsy.

You are thinking of taking up ice skating lessons, but you do not want to injure yourself. Will you be safe to start the lessons whilst the doctors are doing further tests?

Exercise 2

Information for the candidate

Patient details: Mrs Pear, 35 years old

Your role: You are the CMT2 doctor in medical ambulatory care unit.

Please read the referral letter from the patient's GP. You will have 5 minutes to read the letter and take any notes, 14 minutes to take history from the patient, 1 minute to collect your thoughts and 5 minutes with the examiners. You may take your notes with you in the examination room.

Referral letter

Dear Doctor,

Thank you for seeing this lady, who presented with a history of headaches and blurred vision over the last week.

She is otherwise fit and well, and has no other past medical history of note.

I would appreciate your opinion regarding the cause of her headaches and advice on further management.

Kind Regards,

Dr Kelly

Information for the patient

You are Mrs Mary Pear, 35 years old.

Over the last 10 days, you have been having severe headaches. The headache is at the back of your head, and in the front of your head, and it is there constantly.

You never had any headaches in the past as severe as these episodes. This is the worst headache you have had in your life.

It does not wake you up from sleep at night, but you do find it very difficult to go to sleep because the headache gets worse every night. It also gets worse whenever you lie down or bend forward.

You have not vomited with the headache, but you feel nauseated when the pain is very severe. You have not noticed any rashes and you have not noticed any fevers.

You do not get any warning symptoms when the headache is about to get worse, and it basically never leaves you, it is constantly there, but in between the painkillers and if you sneeze or cough, or lie down it gets severely worse.

The only symptom that you have noticed with the headache that is really worrisome is that you think your vision is blurred. You have blurred vision on both eyes during the headaches. Deny any other symptoms asked by the doctor.

You have been taking regular pain killers over the counter, paracetamol and ibuprofen. When you visited your own doctor for stronger pain relief he referred you to the hospital.

Apart from the pain killers, you are also on an oral contraceptive pill, but you take no other medications.

You have smoked 10 cigarettes a day for the last 10 years, and you do not drink alcohol.

You do not have any illnesses, and you used to suffer from migraines as a teenager, but if asked, this headache does not remind you of your migraines.

Your parents are both fit and well. You have no siblings, and you live with your partner. You have no children of your own.

You work as a secretary in an office.

You are really worried whether you have brain cancer. You recently watched a film on TV, when the main actor started having disabling head-aches and he turned out to have cancer.

Your questions to the doctor

What is the diagnosis?

Can they give you stronger pain killers? It is difficult to concentrate on your work when the headache is bad.

Can the headaches be there because of cancer?

Exercise 3

Information for the candidate

Patient details: Mr Orange, 67 years old

Your role: You are the CMT2 doctor in general medical outpatient clinic.

Please read the referral letter from the patient's GP. You will have 5 minutes to read the letter and take any notes, 14 minutes to take history from the patient, 1 minute to collect your thoughts and 5 minutes with the examiners. You may take your notes with you in the examination room.

Referral letter

Dear Doctor,

Thank you for seeing this gentleman, who presented with an ulcer on his left lateral malleolus.

He has diabetes type II, diagnosed 15 years ago, and he is on oral hypoglycaemic agents and insulin. His most recent HbA1c 1 was 64 mmol/mol, 1 month ago.

I would appreciate your opinion regarding the treatment of his ulcer and his diabetes control.

Kind Regards,

Dr Kelly

Information for the patient

You are Mr William Orange, 67 years old.

You were diagnosed with diabetes when you were 55 years old. After an initial period of diet trial, your doctor started you on medications for your diabetes. Despite being on two different medications, your diabetes was not under control, so you have been taking insulin for the last 5 years.

Your sensation in your legs has not been good for years, and you have been told this is because of your diabetes; however, you never had foot ulcers before. You do not wear special shoes. You walk long distances every day, trying to lose weight.

Your wife noticed the foot ulcer a week ago, and this is when you decided to go seek medical help. You have not had any pain.

You have been feeling well and have not had any nausea, fevers, shivers or tiredness.

Your doctor told you that the ulcer may be because of your diabetes. He gave you antibiotics and sent you to hospital to have the ulcer checked.

At the moment, you are on metformin 1 g twice a day, and also insulin: lantus 23 units once a day, in the morning, and also novorapid 6 units three times per day.

You have been trying to lose weight and currently are on a diet. You are not feeling excessively thirsty, and you have not increased urinary frequency, nor urinary symptoms.

Your vision is not very good, and you have had to have laser surgery in both eyes, but you have not noticed any new symptoms for the last 6 months.

You have been instructed to measure your sugars daily, but you do not do that every single day.

You have not been admitted to hospital recently, and the last admission you had was 3 years ago when you had a heart attack.

You have not had a hypoglycaemic episode for years. Last time you had hypoglycaemic episodes was years ago, when you were taking a medication that was subsequently stopped. You have not had any episodes since.

Metformin used to cause you some stomach upset, but not anymore. You take your metformin as you are supposed to, and the same applies to your insulin injections. You are doing the injections in your tummy, and you have had no problems with that.

Your medications are

Metformin, insulin, aspirin, bisoprolol, ramipril, atorvastatin, flucloxacillin. You have no known allergies. You have not taken any other medications, prescribed, or over-the-counter.

You are worried that because of this ulcer, you will not be able to go for regular walks, as advised by your doctor, in order to lose weight.

You have these questions for the doctor

Will you need to come in to hospital?

Is this ulcer going to go away soon?

Why did your doctor give you antibiotics? Is this an infection?

Exercise 4

Information for the candidate

Patient details: Miss Melon, 45 years old

Your role: You are the CMT2 doctor in the general medical outpatient clinic.

Please read the referral letter from the patient's GP. You will have 5 minutes to read the letter and take any notes, 14 minutes to take the history from the patient, 1 minute to collect your thoughts and 5 minutes with the examiners. You may take the notes with you in the examination room.

Referral letter

Dear Doctor,

Thank you for seeing this lady, who was found to have deranged liver function tests during a routine medical exam.

She is otherwise fit and well, and has no other past medical history of note. She does not smoke and drinks alcohol occasionally.

I would appreciate your opinion regarding further investigations and management.

Kind Regards,

Dr Kelly

Information for the patient

You are Mrs Jenny Melon, 45 years old.

You recently had some routine investigations required by your new employer before starting a job as a healthcare practitioner in a private clinic.

You have not had any symptoms, and you were not expecting any blood tests to be abnormal. When you were told that some of your blood tests were abnormal, it came as a shock to you.

The doctor will need to do some further questioning about your general health. If asked specifically, you can volunteer the information below.

You have not noticed any weakness or tiredness, you have not noticed any weight gain or loss. You have not noticed any night sweats, nor hot flushes. You occasionally get headaches. You have been diagnosed with migraines when you were 23 years old, and you get those occasionally. In fact, you have been suffering from attacks for the last month, and you relate that to stress from your recent interview. But the headaches are your usual migraines, and you are not concerned about them. Your bowel habit is not altered and you have not had any nausea or vomiting. Your have not had any urinary symptoms. You have not been getting any palpitations, chest pains or dizziness. You have not noticed any shortness of breath or cough. You have not noticed any bloating, or abdominal distension, and your appetite is good. You have never had any abdominal pains, and you never had a history of gallbladder stones. Neither your family nor you have noticed any discoloration of your skin or eyes. You have not had any bleeding episodes. You have not had any flu-like symptoms recently.

If you are asked about alcohol, you admit to drinking a couple of glasses of wine with your dinner every night. This has been the case for the last couple years. If the doctor insists on questioning you about alcohol, you can admit drinking a bit more than that recently, and you think that is due to stress of the job interview. You do not smoke and never did. You have not travelled abroad recently. You are not on any regular medications. You only take some painkillers over the counter when you have headaches, mainly paracetamol. If asked more details, you have been taking paracetamol almost regularly for the last couple of weeks, but not more than the recommended dose. You have never had any blood transfusions and in fact have never been admitted to hospital. All members of your family are fit and well, and you cannot recall anybody ever having any kind of problems with their liver.

You are worried that these abnormal blood tests may prevent you from getting the job, and you really need the job, as you cannot make ends meet with just your husband's salary.

You have some questions for the doctor

Can these blood tests be abnormal because of alcohol?

Do you need to have more investigations?

Will you need to get admitted to hospital?

Cardiovascular

Aortic stenosis

Presenting a case of *aortic stenosis*

> **Tip!**
> Aortic stenosis is a very common case in PACES, as it is a very common clinical problem, so it is worth knowing inside out! The examiners will expect candidates to perform well, so for top marks, your presentation must be excellent. Aim for full marks on this station.

The three symptoms of aortic stenosis are dyspnoea, angina and syncope, so the synopsis given for a case of aortic stenosis can be:

'This patient presents with shortness of breath, angina symptoms or episodes of syncope. Examine the patient.'

Positive clinical findings

The presentation should be organized on the four categories of presenting a valve disease:

1. *Pulse*: rate, rhythm, character (slow rising if severe), volume; blood pressure
2. *Inspection of the precordium*: for scars
3. *Palpation of the precordium, including apex*: undisplaced apex beat, no heaves, no thrills
4. *Auscultation of the precordium*: ejection systolic murmur; this can extend all the way to S2 if severe.

To achieve full marks within your presentation, after presenting the positive findings leading to your diagnosis, you should comment on possible complications of any valve disease:

- Signs of heart failure, comment on jugular venous pressure (JVP) peripheral oedema, lung bases auscultation
- Stigmata of infective endocarditis; and
- Evidence of anaemia.

Workup

- Twelve lead ECG
- Chest X-ray (CXR)

- Echocardiogram
- Coronary angiogram.

Model presentation

This patient, who presents with episodes of chest pain, is comfortable at rest, with a resting pulse of 70 bpm, regular in rhythm, low in volume and slow-rising in character. There are no scars on inspection of his precordium. The apex beat is not displaced, but it is heaving in character. On auscultation, there is a normal first heart sound, followed by an ejection systolic murmur. The murmur radiates to his carotids, and is best heard on the aortic area in the sitting-up position and on expiration. The second heart sound is also normal.

In summary, this patient has aortic stenosis, which may be the cause of his presenting clinical symptoms.

There are no signs of heart failure, as the lung fields are clear, the JVP is not raised, and there is no peripheral oedema. There are no stigmata of infective endocarditis.

I would like to conclude my examination by performing a full set of observations, including blood pressure and urinalysis.

I would like to obtain a 12-lead ECG to begin, with some baseline blood tests. Then I would proceed to obtain an echocardiogram, so as to confirm my diagnosis and assess the disease severity. Finally, I would refer the patient for a diagnostic coronary angiography to exclude coronary artery disease (CAD) as a cause of his symptoms.

> **MNEMONIC**
>
> Apex in aortic stenosis: *ASH*
>
> **A**ortic **S**tenosis **H**eaving apex

Discussions with the examiners

What investigations are indicated for this patient?

As with every valve problem, the investigations we need are:

- Twelve lead ECG to assess for signs of left ventricular hypertrophy (LVH) and left heart strain—left axis deviation, ST depression in the lateral leads.

- CXR to exclude other diagnosis that could give rise to these kind of symptoms, and assess for cardiomegaly or signs of left ventricular dysfunction, record calcification of the aortic valve and aortic dilation.
- ECHO to confirm diagnosis, exclude other valve problems and estimate severity of stenosis. Echocardiographic criteria for stenosis severity depending on the area of the aortic valve are: the normal area of the aortic valve is around $4\,cm^2$, mild aortic stenosis area $>1.5\,cm^2$, moderate area $1.0–1.5\,cm^2$, and severe aortic stenosis area $<1\,cm^2$. Also, with Doppler studies, the calculated pressure gradient across the valve is very useful in assessing the severity of the aortic stenosis. Pressure gradient more than 50 mmHg means severe aortic stenosis. In addition, the echocardiogram in the context of aortic stenosis is useful in assessing the left ventricular function, which also has to do with the severity of the stenosis itself. Transthoracic echo is frequently all that is required to define the anatomy; however, if poor images are obtained, a transoesophageal scan may be required.
- Coronary angiography to exclude CAD, and also if surgery is indicated, prior to aortic valve replacement (AVR) for coronary artery bypass grafting (CABG) to be performed at the same time. Aortic root measurements can be taken at this time, and if there is any concern regarding the reliability of echo measurements, a pressure gradient can be obtained at cardiac catheterization.

How would you manage this patient?

If the patient's synopsis refers to a specific symptom that can be caused by aortic stenosis (i.e. chest pains, syncopal episodes during exercise or dyspnoea), then AVR has to be considered first, as one of the indications of AVR is symptomatic stenosis. Remember that prior to the operation, a coronary angiogram has to be performed to look for coexistent CAD.

So, if asked by the examiners how you would proceed to manage this patient, who presents with the above symptoms, after listing your investigations, you should mention that he needs referral to a specialist service of cardiology/cardiothoracic multi-disciplinary team (MDT) for discussion for possible AVR on the grounds that he is symptomatic.

However, the general management of aortic stenosis is:

- Regular followup with clinical examination and yearly echocardiograms, if the patient is free of symptoms, and there are no criteria of severe stenosis in the echocardiogram. Cautious control of hypertension and cardiac risk factor management.

- Dental prophylaxis is not currently recommended by NICE.
- AVR in symptomatic patients, or severe aortic stenosis in echocardiography, or in the event that the patient has severe CAD, that CABG is indicated as a treatment option.
- For those unfit to undergo open AVR, TAVI (transcatheter aortic valve intervention) is a possible option.

What are the complications of aortic stenosis?

Aortic stenosis results in pressure overload to the left ventricle, which causes ventricular hypertrophy, and can give rise to left ventricular failure, as well as ventricular arrhythmias. Inadequate cardiac output because of arrhythmia or the stenosis itself can lead to syncope or sudden death. If the cause of the stenosis is degenerative calcification, valve apparatus disintegration can cause embolic episodes. Infective endocarditis can be a complication of any valve disease. Also, in aortic stenosis, an acquired defect in von Willebrand factor may occur, giving rise to bleeding diathesis, usually presenting with gastrointestinal bleeding.

MNEMONIC

Complications: LE_2A_2P

Left ventricular failure
Endocarditis
Emboli
Anaemia
Arrhythmias
Pulmonary hypertension

Aortic regurgitation

Presenting a case of *aortic regurgitation*

Tip!

Chronic aortic regurgitation is well compensated by left ventricular dilation as a response to volume load, so patients are usually asymptomatic until the lesion is well advanced.

For the above reason, the synopsis for aortic regurgitation usually is:

'This patient was found to have a murmur. Please examine them.'

Positive clinical findings

Again start your presentation by commenting on the four categories of clinical signs plus two categories of signs presenting as complications:

1. *Pulse*: collapsing radial pulse, look for vigorous carotid pulsations (representing the wide pulse pressure, Corrigan's pulse)
2. *Inspection*: no scars on the precordium, no head nodding (De Musset's sign) or pulsations in the nail bed (area under the fingernail turns pink-white with each heartbeat, Quincke's sign)
3. *Palpation*: apex beat is displaced laterally (as in all regurgitations of the left heart valves), and it is thrusting (representing hyperdynamic circulation)
4. *Auscultation*: early diastolic murmur loudest at the lower left sternal edge on expiration, when patient is sitting forward.

There are (no) signs of heart failure and there are (no) stigmata of endocarditis.

Offer to measure blood pressure in both arms, paying close attention to the pulse pressure and any differential.

> ### Tip!
> Remember collapsing pulse and thrusting apex beat both represent hyperdynamic circulation. All states that can result in hyperdynamic circulation can give the same signs, e.g. thyrotoxicosis, anaemia, pregnancy, fever.

It is also important to be alert for clinical signs suggestive of Marfan's syndrome, or other connective tissue disorder, which are commonly associated with aortic valve incompetence.

Workup

*   Twelve lead ECG (for PR interval, signs of LVH or strain).
*   Transthoracic echo (to confirm the diagnosis with Doppler studies, determine a possible cause and assess the valve and the left ventricle).

- Transoesophageal echo may be needed (to assess the valve in more detail, especially where bicuspid valve, endocarditis or coexistent disease of another valve is suspected); however, in many cases, excellent images of the aortic valve can be obtained via the transthoracic route alone.
- Coronary angiogram (if CAD is suspected, or if AVR is an option, prior to the surgery, to assess whether CABG is indicated at the same time, aortic root measurements can be taken at this time).
- Aortic CT or MRI (is sometimes indicated to assess aortic root size).

Model presentation

This patient is comfortable at rest, with a resting pulse of 70 beats per minute, regular in rhythm, of large volume. The carotid pulsations are even visible from the bedside, and of a collapsing character. On inspection of his precordium there are no scars, and on palpation of his precordium, there are no palpable heaves or thrills, but the apex beat is displaced laterally, and is thrusting.

On auscultation, there is a diastolic murmur, better heard at the left sternal edge, which is loudest when the patient is sitting forward and on expiration.

There are no signs of heart failure, as the lung fields are clear, the JVP is not raised, and there is no peripheral oedema. There are no peripheral stigmata of infective endocarditis.

In summary, the murmur that was identified in this patient is due to aortic regurgitation.

I would like to complete my examination by looking at his observation chart and his urine dipstick, and I would proceed with a 12-lead ECG and an echocardiogram in the first instance.

> **Tip!**
> Other murmurs that can be heard in aortic regurgitation are:
> - mid-diastolic in the apex, due to functional mitral stenosis (Austin Flint murmur) and
> - ejection systolic in the aortic area (flow murmur), due to increased volume of blood through the aortic valve.

So, if you make a spot diagnosis of the above, you may want to present your case in a different way.

Model presentation if spot diagnosis of a specific phenotype is made

This young patient has phenotype features of Marfan's syndrome. On examination, his pulse is 70 bpm, regular, and collapsing in character, and I can note vigorous carotid pulsations in his neck. There are no scars on the precordium. On palpation of his precordium, the apex beat is displaced and thrusting in quality. There is also a diastolic murmur at the left sternal edge, with normal first and second heart sounds.

In summary, this patient's murmur is due to aortic regurgitation, probably related to Marfan's syndrome.

There are no signs of pulmonary hypertension or heart failure, and there are no stigmata of infective endocarditis.

I would like to complete my examination by obtaining a full set of observations, including blood pressure and urinalysis, and perform a more detailed examination to look for specific signs associated with aortic regurgitation.

I would request an echocardiogram in the first instance to confirm my diagnosis, assess regurgitation severity, look for other valve problems and assess ventricular function. Depending on the echocardiogram results, I would decide on further investigations and referral to cardiology outpatients.

MNEMONIC

Apex in aortic regurgitation: *AORTA*

Aortic **R**egurgitation
Thrusting **A**pex

Discussion with the examiners

What are the causes of aortic regurgitation?

Acute aortic regurgitation can be caused by aortic dissection, ruptured aneurysms, or infective endocarditis; however, in PACES exam, the case will represent chronic aortic regurgitation, as the patient has to be stable enough to take part in the exams. In chronic aortic regurgitation, the causes are many. Listing some of them is appropriate in the exams.

> **MNEMONIC**
>
> Causes of aortic regurgitation: *PRIMA*
>
> - **P**rosthetic valve not working well (in which case presentation has to be according to AVR)
> - **R**heumatoid arthritis
> - **R**heumatic fever
> - **I**nfective endocarditis
> - **M**arfan and other connective tissue disorders
> - **A**nkylosing spondylitis and other causes of aortitis

How would you proceed with this patient?

Echocardiography remains the mainstay of investigation and followup in aortic regurgitation. Patients should be seen annually and examined for evidence of heart failure, assessment of blood pressure and to ensure no signs of endocarditis. An ECG should be performed at every visit (PR interval, LVH). Echo in asymptomatic patients should be at least once every 2 years.

Medical management consists of followup, control of hypertension with vasodilators (ACE inhibitors or ARBs) and cardiac risk factors, regular dental checkups and any work necessary. Beta blockers may worsen symptoms as they prolong diastole; however, there is some evidence that they slow the rate of aortic root dilatation in Marfan's syndrome.

Indications for surgery are symptomatic patients (syncope, heart failure symptoms), LV ejection fraction below 50%, patients undergoing other cardiac surgery (e.g. CABG), LV dilatation (end diastolic diameter >70 mm). Marfan's or bicuspid valve patients should have surgery when aortic root diameter is 50 mm or greater, others at 55 mm. The European Society of Cardiology publishes comprehensive guidance on the management of valvular heart disease.

Mitral regurgitation

How to present a case of *mitral regurgitation*

Mitral regurgitation can cause heart failure and atrial fibrillation (AF) because of atrial dilation due to the volume overload. So the synopsis can be:

'This patient complains of shortness of breath or palpitations. Please examine the patient.'

Positive clinical findings

1. *Pulse*: irregularly irregular (if in AF)
2. *Inspection*: if left lateral thoracotomy scar, patient had previous valvotomy
3. *Palpation*: apex is displaced and thrusting (as in all regurgitations of left heart because of hyperdynamic circulation), present parasternal heave/thrill
4. *Auscultation*: pansystolic murmur loudest at the apex, on expiration at the left lateral position, radiating to the axilla.

> **Tip!**
> All mitral valve diseases (whether stenosis or regurgitation or mixed valve disease) can be complicated with atrial arrhythmias and specifically AF. So beware, when identifying irregularly irregular pulse, a mitral valve pathology might be coming.

> **Tip!**
> All regurgitations of the left heart (aortic or mitral) can cause displacement of the apex beat laterally.

Having diagnosed mitral regurgitation, it is important to comment on signs of *pulmonary hypertension*.

Remember the volume load goes backwards, causing volume load to the pulmonary arteries and the right heart.

These signs are loud pulmonary component of the second heart sound, raised JVP with prominent V waves.

If the pulmonary hypertension has caused tricuspid and pulmonary regurgitation, the associated murmurs can be heard:

- Pansystolic murmur at the left lower sternal edge (tricuspid regurgitation)
- Early diastolic murmur at the left upper sternal edge (pulmonary regurgitation).

> ### Tip!
> In all mitral valve lesions, look specifically for signs of pulmonary hypertension:
> - Loud P2
> - Raised JVP with big V waves in the neck
> - Left parasternal heave/thrill
> - Pansystolic murmur of tricuspid regurgitation and diastolic murmur of pulmonary regurgitation.

Model presentation

This patient is comfortable at rest with a resting pulse of 60 bpm, irregularly irregular. On inspection of his precordium, there are no scars. On palpation, the apex beat is displaced laterally, with an apical thrill. On auscultation, the first heart sound is soft, followed by a pansystolic murmur, best heard in the apex, in the left lateral position, and in expiration. It radiates to the axilla. There are no signs of heart failure.

In summary, this patient has mitral regurgitation.

The lung fields are clear, there are no signs of pulmonary hypertension, and no stigmata of infective endocarditis.

I would like to finish my examination by obtaining a full set of observations, including blood pressure and urinalysis.

Workup

- Twelve lead ECG
- CXR
- Echocardiogram
- Consider diagnostic coronary angiography.

Discussion with the examiners

What other lesions can give rise to a pansystolic murmur?
- Tricuspid regurgitation
- Ventricular septal defect (VSD).

What are the causes of mitral regurgitation?
Organize these into three categories:
- Acute mitral regurgitation (MR) is seen in the context of myocardial infarction (papillary muscle or chordae tendonae rupture), infective endocarditis.

- Functional MR occurs when there is left ventricular dilatation, which stretches the mitral annulus so that the two leaflets don't meet when they close (the valve itself is usually normal in these cases). This is usually due to ischaemic heart disease, dilated cardiomyopathy or hypertension.
- Chronic MR is due to valve calcification (degenerative), rheumatic fever or connective tissue disease. Mitral valve prolapse and congenital MR can also cause chronic MR.

How would you advise this patient regarding dental treatment?

Routine antibiotic prophylaxis is not currently recommended by NICE for valvular heart disease; however, the dentist should be made aware of the presence of valve disease. The patient should undergo regular dental inspections and prophylactic repair work as necessary to reduce the risk of abscess formation. Patients on warfarin should have this managed for any operative procedure.

How would you investigate this patient further?

- As with all valvular heart disease, clinical examination and echocardiography is the mainstay of investigation and followup.
- Serial ECGs should be taken to look for the development of AF, and a CXR is useful to look for signs of pulmonary congestion and infection.
- For chronic MR, at each visit, the patient should be examined for signs of heart failure and pulmonary hypertension. Increasing breathlessness or decreasing exercise tolerance may signal either the onset of AF or worsening regurgitation and may be a trigger to consider intervention.
- Transthoracic echocardiography can be used to visualize the valve anatomy, measure the size of the left atrium and ventricle, quantify the degree of regurgitation and estimate pulmonary artery pressure. As the mitral valve is a posterior structure, however, in some patients the image quality may be poor and transoesophageal echo is needed for a more accurate assessment.
- Transoesophageal echo is routinely used to assess suitability for surgery, and is also performed intra-operatively.
- Cardiac catheterization is used to assess for CAD in those under consideration for valve surgery (CABG can be performed at the same time). Right heart catheterization is often also performed to assess pulmonary pressure, and left ventriculography is infrequently used nowadays as it can precipitate pulmonary oedema.

How would you manage this patient?

Patients should be followed up at regular intervals, with echo annually, or twice yearly if there is concern about rapid deterioration.

Heart failure should be managed conventionally, with consideration of surgery. In cases of LV dilatation causing functional MR, treating the underlying cause may allow the valve lesion to regress.

Dental health as described above should be monitored.

Patients who develop AF are at high risk for embolic complications and should be anticoagulated. Warfarin is licensed for this, and recent trials have demonstrated new oral anticoagulants (NOACs) (such as dabigatran, rivaroxaban and apixiban) to be inferior and should not be used.

Surgical intervention for MR includes valve replacement or repair (in favourable cases), which is usually done as open surgery. If annular dilatation is the cause, this can be repaired when medical therapy to reduce LV dilatation is not an option (a percutaneous approach has been tried, but is not currently available in the United Kingdom).

What are the possible causes of mitral regurgitation?

CAUSES OF MITRAL REGURGITATION

PRIDE

- **P**rolapsed mitral valve
- **R**heumatic heart and rheumatoid arthritis
- **I**schaemic heart disease
- **D**egenerative calcification
- **E**ndocarditis

Rheumatic fever is uncommon in the United Kingdom; however, it remains prevalent in developing countries. Similarly, acute MR due to ruptured papillary muscle or chordae is less common in the era of primary percutaneous coronary intervention where revascularization is prompt, however, in those with delayed presentation of myocardial infarction it is sometimes still seen. It typically occurs 72 h–2 weeks post-infarct, and the differential diagnosis is acute VSD.

Mitral stenosis

Presenting a case of *mitral stenosis*

Mitral stenosis can give rise to a variety of symptoms, but the most common synopsis for this case will be:

'This patient is complaining of shortness of breath/tiredness. Please examine the patient.'

Alternative, common presentations will include palpitations, recent onset AF and frequent chest infections (especially left-sided pneumonia).

Positive clinical findings

Your presentation should follow the order below, as with all valve problems:
1. *Pulse*: normal in character (as all mitral problems), irregularly irregular (if in AF)
2. *Inspection*: no scars, may have malar flush
3. *Palpation*: nondisplaced apex (as in all stenosis), tapping (tapping apex you will find on any case producing loud first heart sound), no heaves or thrills (as in all stenosis)

> **Tip!**
> Stenosed valves do not cause a displaced apex. Only regurgitation across the valves causes volume overload, and thus displaces the apex beat. Stenosis of the valves, on the contrary, causes pressure overload.

4. *Auscultation*: loud S_1 with normal S_2; there is an opening snap in diastole, followed by a mid-diastolic murmur with presystolic accentuation (if patient is in sinus rhythm).

To achieve full marks within your presentation, you should comment on the presence or absence of complications.

Mitral stenosis can give rise to many symptoms and a number of complications, and that is why it is very important, when you have identified such a diagnosis, to comment on important negatives on examination.

MNEMONIC

Complications of Mitral stenosis (MS): *ATROPIne*

Atrial fibrillation

Thromboembolic disease

Right heart failure

Oedema (pulmonary and peripheral)

Pulmonary hypertension

Infective endocarditis

Workup

- Twelve lead ECG (p mitrale, AF, right ventricular hypertrophy)
- Echocardiogram (to confirm diagnosis and assess the severity, LV function and LA size, pulmonary artery pressure)
- CXR (signs of heart failure, double silhouette from left atrium enlargement)
- Cardiac catheterization and coronary angiography (in selected patients, for example prior to valve replacement).

Model presentation

This patient is comfortable at rest, with a resting pulse of 70 beats per minute, irregularly irregular. On inspection of his precordium, there are no scars. On palpation, the apex beat is not displaced, and there are no heaves or thrills. On auscultation, the first heart sound is loud. There is an opening snap in diastole, followed by a mid-diastolic murmur in the apex.

In summary, this patient has mitral stenosis, which is complicated by AF.

There are no signs of right or left heart failure, as there is no peripheral oedema, JVP is not raised and the lung fields are clear. There are no signs of pulmonary hypertension either. There are no stigmata of endocarditis.

I would like to finish my examination by obtaining a full set of observations, including blood pressure and urinalysis. I would specifically ask this patient about a history of rheumatic fever.

I would like to perform a 12-lead ECG to confirm that this patient is in AF, and an echocardiogram to confirm the finding of mitral stenosis, as well as assess the degree of severity, and the ventricular function. Other important findings will be the LA size and pulmonary artery pressure. I would then proceed to cardiac catheterization to exclude CAD as the cause of his symptoms.

Workup

- Twelve lead ECG
- Echocardiogram (transthoracic in the first instance, but a transoesophageal is often required to fully assess the mitral valve)
- CXR
- Coronary angiography.

Discussion with the examiners

What are other differentials of a mid-diastolic murmur with the above characteristics?
- Atrial myxoma
- Atrial thrombus.

What are the causes of mitral stenosis?
Rheumatic fever is the predominant cause of mitral stenosis, although this is uncommonly seen in the United Kingdom. Other causes include carcinoid syndrome, congenital defects and prosthetic valve dysfunction.

How would you investigate this patient?
- The ECG is the initial test you would order in any patient with cardiovascular symptomatology. In this case, you would be able to assess for atrial arrhythmias, which are very common with mitral valve pathologies, as well as obtain some indirect information about the left atrium and left ventricle.
- A CXR should always be requested. Specific findings to look for include cardiomegaly, left atrial dilatation and pulmonary congestion or infection.
- Echocardiogram is a very important tool in any valve pathology. Apart from confirming your diagnosis, it will help you quantify the severity of the stenosis with objective measures, and inform you about the function of the other valves and the ventricles. The mitral valve is often poorly seen via transthoracic imaging, so a transoesophageal study is often required to assess in more detail, especially in cases where a surgical repair of the valve is considered. Stress echocardiography is used to assess further when there is a mismatch between symptoms and severity by echo.
- If the patient needs valve replacement, or if he has presented with symptoms that can be caused by CAD, a diagnostic coronary angiography is the next investigation.

How would you manage this patient?

- If the patient is asymptomatic, and in sinus rhythm, then regular followup with clinical examination, symptom enquiry and yearly echocardiograms are the only requirements. Deterioration can be rapid, often precipitated by AF.
- If the patient has developed AF, then assessment for the need of formal anticoagulation is needed, as well as control of the underlying ventricular rate.

> **Tip!**
> Remember that all the NOACs have been studied and gained approval only in the context of nonvalvular AF, so avoid mentioning them in a case of mitral stenosis.

- If the patient has developed symptoms of heart failure, then appropriate treatment should be initiated both for prognostic benefit and symptom control.
- Intervention is indicated when the valve area is <1.5 cm^2, in severe mitral stenosis, symptomatology of pulmonary hypertension or recurrent emboli. Percutaneous valvuloplasty is preferred if there is no CAD, no valve calcification, no additional mitral regurgitation, no thrombus formation and the leaflets are mobile. Otherwise, mitral valve replacement (MVR) is preferred. Mitral valve repair may be suitable for a small number of selected patients.

How can you explain the different symptoms and complication of mitral stenosis?

In mitral stenosis, the left atrium becomes pressure-overloaded and in time dilates. This can cause atrial arrhythmias, most commonly AF. The increased pressure is transmitted backwards to the pulmonary system, causing pulmonary hypertension, dyspnoea, orthopnoea, pulmonary oedema, and due to chronically excessive fluid extravasation, haemoptysis and recurrent chest infections. The enlarged left atrium can also compress the left main bronchus, leading to stasis pneumonia. Because of the AF, these patients can have embolic episodes (strokes), and because sometimes the enlarged atrium presses the laryngeal nerve, it can lead to Ortner's syndrome (dysphonia). Chronic pulmonary hypertension results in right heart failure, resulting in peripheral oedema, hepatomegaly, ascites and raised JVP.

Also, because of mitral stenosis, the cardiac output is reduced, resulting in fatigue, tiredness, shortness of breath, reduced exercise tolerance and malar flush.

What is the medical treatment for this patient?

Although intervention is the primary treatment of mitral stenosis, diuretics, nitrates, beta blockers and anticoagulants may all play a role in the symptomatic management. It is worth noting that many patients will be female and of child-bearing age, which affects greatly upon the timing of any intervention (pregnancy can cause a stable patient to deteriorate rapidly) and the use of anticoagulants. Long-term followup with clinical examination and echocardiography is required even after intervention.

Prosthetic valve replacements

Presenting a case of a *prosthetic valve*

Positive clinical findings

Go through your positive findings in the order that you have been following for presenting valve disease:

1. *Pulse*: character, volume, rhythm, rate.
2. *Inspection of the precordium*: midline sternotomy scar. When you see a midline sternotomy scar, look for:
   a. Surgical graft scars in the limbs, as patients might have had valve replacement and CABG.
   b. At the same time, also look for thoracotomy scar on the left, which represents minimally invasive mitral valve surgery.
   c. Check to ensure the scars are well healed and look healthy.
   d. Additional small scars may be seen on epigastrium from surgical drain and pacing wires placed at the time of the operation.
3. *Palpation of the precordium*: comment on apex, and presence of heaves and thrills.
4. *Auscultation*: prominent S1 in MVR, prominent S2 in AVR, click coinciding with S1 in mechanical MVR, click coinciding with S2 in AVR.

> **Tip!**
> A bioprosthetic valve will have a distinct click to it. Beware of other murmurs as patients will often have multiple valve pathologies. Also be aware of bivalve replacements.

> **Tip!**
>
> With a mechanical prosthetic valve, you can hear an audible click even before using the stethoscope, as you are feeling for the carotid pulse. If the audible click coincides with the pulse, it is a MVR; if the audible click follows the pulse, it is an AVR.

> **Tip!**
>
> In MVR, look for a left lateral thoracotomy scar, which reveals previous valvotomy for mitral stenosis.

Presence of complications

MNEMONIC

Complications of valve replacement: *HATED*

Haemolysis/haemorrhage (look for signs of anaemia)
Anticoagulation side effects (look for purpura)
Thromboembolism
Endocarditis (look for stigmata)
Dysfunction of the valve (new murmurs, thrombosis, heart failure)

> **Tip!**
>
> In MVR, look specifically for signs of pulmonary hypertension:
> - Loud P2
> - Raised JVP with big V waves in the neck
> - Left parasternal heave/thrill
> - Pansystolic murmur of tricuspid regurgitation and diastolic murmur of pulmonary regurgitation.

Workup
- Detailed history of patient's symptoms
- Urinalysis and blood tests, including blood cultures
- Twelve lead ECG

- Echocardiogram (TTE/TOE)
- Possible angiography.

Model presentation

This 76-year-old gentleman is comfortable at rest, with a resting pulse of 70 beats per minute and regular. On inspection of his precordium, there is a healthy looking, well healed midline sternotomy scar, and on palpation there are no heaves or thrills and the apex beat is not displaced. There are no other scars identified. On auscultation, there is a normal first heart sound, followed by a soft ejection systolic murmur that does not radiate to the carotids, and there is a prosthetic click coinciding with the second heart sound.

There are no peripheral stigmata of infective endocarditis. There are no signs of heart failure, as the lung fields are clear, JVP is not raised and there is no peripheral oedema.

The patient is not clinically anaemic. The patient must be receiving therapeutic anticoagulation, as there is evident purpura on his limbs.

In summary, this patient has a mechanical AVR, which appears to be functioning well.

I would like to complete my examination by measuring the patient's blood pressure, dipstick his urine and perform a full set of observations.

I would like to obtain a full detailed history of the patient's symptoms and proceed to a 12-lead ECG and blood tests. I would also like to request an echocardiogram to assess his valve and ventricular function.

> **Tip!**
> Beware the double valve replacement—mixed signs of AVR and MVR.

Discussion with the examiners

What investigations would you request for this patient?

> **Tip!**
> When you list your investigations during the exam, you should justify why you want to request each investigation that you list. The examiners need to know that you have a rationale for investigating a patient. Do not just list investigations without providing a reason as to why you do them.

The patient will have a presenting complaint related to cardiovascular pathology. The possibilities include:

'This patient presents with … shortness of breath/chest pains/palpitations/ dizzy spells/syncopal episodes.'

The examiners are marking you for correct diagnosis and differential diagnosis. If your presentation for this station is adequate or excellent, you will achieve a satisfactory outcome for this section. The next clinical domains they are marking you on are clinical judgment and appropriate investigations. In order for them to mark you as satisfactory in this section, the examiners need to know that you can correlate your clinical findings and the clinical picture of the patient with a list of appropriate investigations to support your diagnosis and decide on further management. As with all cardiology cases, the first investigation you need is an ECG, as it will give you information for both structural heart problems and arrhythmias that can give rise to all the symptoms listed in the synopsis above. You also need a CXR to assess the lung fields. Before referral to a specialist, you also need an echocardiogram, as with all cardiology cases, on this occasion, to assess for valve and ventricular function. Transthoracic echo is the initial first-line modality, but eventually a transoesophageal echo may be needed, especially for assessing a mitral prosthetic valve, and investigating for endocarditis. Depending on the presenting complaint on your synopsis given for the patient, angiography may be indicated.

> **Tip!**
> Although you are in a CVS station, remember the examiners need to know that you can act as a registrar and think outside the box. If a patient presents with dyspnoea, although you are asked to examine his cardiovascular system, a respiratory pathology can still give rise to such a clinical presentation.

How would you manage this patient?

The next thing the examiners will ask you is how you would manage this patient. The answer here has to include two elements:

- Firstly, based on your working diagnosis, how would you treat this patient's symptoms?
- Secondly, you should say you would refer this patient to a specialty clinic where further investigations may be organized based on the initial results.

Management of the postoperative valve patient includes long-term followup, anticoagulation management and vigilance for endocarditis, arrhythmias (AF is common in mitral valve patients, heart block in aortic valve patients), anaemia and heart failure.

What are the pros and cons of different types of valves?

Tip!		
Valve type	Indications	Pros/cons
Bioprosthetic • Bovine/porcine	Aortic valve >65-year-old patients Mitral valve >70-year-old patients	• No need for long-term anticoagulation, just for 1–3 months postop • Calcification over time
Mechanical • Bileaflet • Cage ball • Tilting disc	Younger patients	• Longer life • Requires lifelong anticoagulation Target INR: Aortic 2–3 Mitral 2.5–3.5

Who would you refer this patient to following initial investigations?

Depending on what the working diagnosis is, whether this patient is developing new signs of heart failure or shows signs of valve dysfunction, he should be referred to a cardiology department in the first instance.

Normally, following valve replacement, patients are followed up by
• cardiothoracic surgeons postoperatively and
• cardiologists annually with transthoracic echocardiogram (echo is not necessarily needed in mechanic valves, or for the first 5 years in bioprosthetic valves, unless symptoms arise).

A referral to the cardiology services is appropriate initially, and the patient may or may not need discussion within a cardiology/cardiothoracic MDT.

If this patient is listed to have an elective total hip replacement, what advice would you give to the orthopaedic team regarding anticoagulation?

- Management of anticoagulated valve in patients undergoing noncardiac surgery/procedures: All trusts should have a 'bridging' policy in place. In brief, low bleeding risk procedures should continue anticoagulation uninterrupted. Medium/high bleed risk usually involves stopping warfarin 1 week prior, therapeutic low molecular weight heparin (LMWH) coverup until the night before surgery, then reintroduction of warfarin 1–2 days postop. If asked by the examiners, but you do not remember the exact details, you should answer that you would consult local policy and seek advice. MVR patients are at a higher thrombotic risk than AVR. Do not panic if you do not remember specific protocols during the exam; the examiners would never mark you down for that.

- Management of bleeding in a mechanical valve patient will require specialist input from cardiology/cardiothoracics and possibly haematology. Anticoagulation should be reversed in life-threatening bleeding after specialist advice.

- NICE no longer recommends prophylactic antibiotics for valve patients undergoing surgical/endoscopic/dental procedures. Other bodies differ in their opinion.

Where to find patients for practise

The best place to find valve replacement cases is the cardiothoracic/cardiology outpatient clinic where patients with valve replacements will have their followup. Valve replacements are easy to diagnose in PACES exam, so having examined six patients with AVR and six patients with MVR is an adequate number for you to spot all the signs needed to prepare.

> **Tip!**
> Visit the cardiothoracic wards to find preop patients admitted the night before operation and postop patients in recovery.
> Most hospitals will also now have specific valve followup clinics.

Central nervous system

Presenting and diagnosing neurology cases

In neurology cases in PACES examination, the most important thing to remember is that usually the examination and diagnosis of a case are all about pattern recognition and formulating the site of the pathology.

Usually, the synopsis of the patient would ask you to examine the lower limbs or the upper limbs or the cranial nerves. But in cases of 'look and approach', like in a patient with hemiplegia, or Parkinson's disease (PD), the synopsis might be more general, as 'examine the patient's neurology system'.

In cases of general guidance based on the patient's synopsis, if you identify early what diagnosis or presentation you have to deal with, you can be guided accordingly to perform a more focused neurological examination, rather than a full one, as you won't have time for the latter.

Although neurology is the station that trainees fear the most amongst the clinical stations, the reality is that it is the simplest clinical station in PACES examination, as it does not rely on your senses but on your technique. If you employ a good examination technique, you will discover the findings that are present and that will enable you to formulate a diagnosis without difficulty. All you have to do is present your positive findings as you identified them, and the diagnosis will be easy to figure out; however, you have to trust your examination skills and ability to interpret what you identify; do not doubt your findings, as this may leave you struggling to get the diagnosis.

The only thing you will be called to do is put the findings together to form either a diagnosis or a differential list. In some cases, it is impossible to give a single diagnosis, in which case the examiners expect you to come up with a list of differential diagnoses; however, it is worth noting that when you give a list of differential diagnoses, present only one to three of the most likely conditions or diagnoses that fit with your findings in the case and demographic of the patient (e.g. age and gender). After reading this chapter, the task of putting the findings together should be an easy achievement.

In this chapter, we have tried to categorize the different cases that appear in PACES. Here are the most commonly presenting cases, with their characteristic physical findings from the neurology examinations.

The most common cases in this station are:

Specific diagnosis cases

1. Multiple sclerosis (MS)
2. Charcot–Marie–Tooth (CMT) (hereditary motor sensory neuropathy)

3. Motor neurone disease (MND)
4. Myotonic dystrophy (MD)
5. PD

Patterns that need differentials

1. Peripheral neuropathy
2. Cerebellar syndrome
3. Spastic paraparesis
4. Hemiparesis, hemiplegia
5. Wasting of the small muscles of the hand

The synopsis for these cases can vary, depending on which part of the neurology system examiners want to guide you to concentrate on. That would probably be the part of the neurology examination that has the most positive findings for the exam. Usually the synopsis would be, 'This patient is complaining of difficulty walking. Please examine their peripheral nervous system (PNS).'

SPECIFIC DIAGNOSIS CASES

Multiple sclerosis

Positive clinical findings

> **Tip!**
> MS cases can have a wide range of combination of signs. Remember that if you have identified multiple signs from different parts of your examination, see if you can put them all together to fit a pattern of MS presentation.

The possible mixture of findings are:
1. cerebellar (dysarthria, nystagmus, ataxia, dysdiadochokinesis, impaired pinpoint testing, intention tremor),
2. pyramidal (loss of power in the limbs with hypertonia and increased reflexes),
3. dorsal column (loss of proprioception and vibration impaired with other modalities of sensation intact),

4. brainstem (internuclear opthalmoplegia) and
5. optic nerve (atrophy of the optic disc in fundoscopy, relative afferent pupillary defect).

Your patient does not need to have all of them. Any combination of the above patterns should raise the suspicion of demyelinating disease, and the presentation should conclude with MS as the diagnosis.

MNEMONIC

Combination of signs of MS: *I COPD*

*I*nternuclear ophthalmoplegia
*C*erebellar
*O*ptic nerve
*P*yramidal weakness
*D*orsal column signs

Model presentation

Lower limbs

On examination of her lower limbs, this patient has bilateral pyramidal weakness, with hypertonia and hyperreflexia, more marked on the left side. There is also bilateral ataxia of her lower limbs, with loss of coordination, with impaired heel-shin testing. Testing of her lower limb sensation revealed loss of vibration and proprioception bilaterally. Both of her plantars are upgoing. Her gait is broad-based and ataxic, and she is using walking aids.

In summary, this lady presents with a combination of cerebellar corticospinal tract and dorsal column signs in her lower limbs. The most likely diagnosis is demyelinating disease, such as MS.

Upper limbs

This patient has pyramidal weakness of her right upper limb, with hypertonia and hyperreflexia. There is also ataxia on the same upper limb, with dysdiadochokinesis and intention tremor. She has also loss of vibration sensation and proprioception in her upper limbs bilaterally.

In summary, this lady presents with a combination of cerebellar corticospinal tract and dorsal column signs in her lower limbs. The most likely diagnosis is demyelinating disease, such as MS.

Cranial nerves

On examination of her eyes, this patient has internuclear ophthalmoplegia and bilateral nystagmus with hypermetric saccades. On fundoscopy, the right optic disc is atrophic. She also displays right-sided facial weakness of upper motor neurone origin.

In summary, this patient has a combination of optic atrophy and brainstem signs in her cranial nerve examination, and demyelinating disease is on the top of my differential list. I would also like to examine her PNS to look for cerebellar, dorsal column and spinal cord signs.

No matter what the initial synopsis is for such a patient, if you have time during the exam, do proceed to perform a focused exam to demonstrate other signs that will reveal MS. For example, if the synopsis asks you to examine this patient's lower limbs, and you demonstrate pyramidal and cerebellar signs, with loss of vibration, you can proceed to test the eyes and the fundi, as the more signs you can put together, the more your diagnosis is certain, and the examiners will also be reassured that you know what to look for in such a case.

Discussion with the examiners

How would you confirm your diagnosis on this patient?

- *Clinical suspicion*: the diagnosis of MS is a clinical one.
- *Brain and spinal cord imaging*: MRI is the investigation of choice to support the clinical diagnosis.
- The diagnosis consists of the confirmation of lesions that disseminate in time and place.
- *Cerebrospinal fluid (CSF) analysis*: lumbar puncture can help the diagnosis with the demonstration of oligoclonal bands in the CSF.
- *Evoked potentials*: may be helpful in identifying the site of a lesion that is not apparent in initial imaging.

How would you treat this patient?

- *Multidisciplinary approach*: many healthcare professionals need to get involved in the management of MS, including physiotherapists, neurologists, occupational therapists and psychologists.
- *Patient education*: patient's education about their disease, the potential progression and the prognosis is essential and especially important if the initial diagnosis involves a young woman of childbearing age.
- *Treat the acute attacks*: acute attacks that cause neurological compromise need urgent attention, possible hospitalization and treatment with steroids, either intravenously or orally.

- *Specific treatments*: in relapsing remitting pattern of MS, there are specific therapies, such as interferon-β, that have been used for years, as well as newer agents, taken orally, that do not treat MS, but have shown to slow progression in some cases.

Hereditary sensory and motor neuropathy

> **Tip!**
> This is a very common case in PACES exam. The most common synopsis will ask you to examine the patient's lower limbs, as the relevant findings will be more obvious in the legs; however, when you finish the lower limb examination, if time allows, you can proceed to examine the upper limbs briefly, looking for the same findings, as the same process also affects the upper limbs.

Positive clinical findings

The characteristic findings you will elicit are:

1. *distal wasting*: this is what gives the legs the 'inverted champagne bottle' appearance;
2. *distal weakness*: in severe cases of long-standing disease, patients may have some element of proximal weakness as well; however, that would not be as marked as the distal weakness, especially foot dorsiflexion;
3. *distal sensation reduced*: all modalities and
4. reflexes and plantars absent.

Model presentation

This patient has evident bilateral symmetrical distal motor and sensory neuropathy. On inspection of his lower limbs, there is distal wasting, bilateral pes cavus and clawing of his toes.

On examination of power, there is bilateral and symmetrical distal weakness of his lower limbs with bilateral foot drop.

On examination of his reflexes, both the tendon reflexes as well as plantar responses are absent.

On examination of his sensation, all modalities of sensation are reduced distally.

His gait is high stoppage and ataxic.

In summary, this patient has long-standing distal motor and sensory neuropathy in his lower limbs. All these signs favour a diagnosis of CMT disease.

> **Tip!**
> When you have identified a peripheral sensorimotor neuropathy, try to identify:
> 1. If there are clinical signs that suggest chronicity; if they are present, then in most probability, this disease is long-standing, thus a hereditary cause rather than an acquired one should be your initial diagnosis.
> 2. If there are features/evidence of tests, like scars from nerve biopsies, do comment on them on your presentation.

I would like to proceed with my examination by testing the upper limbs to see whether the same process is affecting his hands.

Discussion with the examiners

How would you confirm your diagnosis?
The diagnosis can be confirmed with nerve conduction studies, genetic testing and nerve biopsy.

- Nerve conduction studies will show decreased velocity if the problem is demyelination.
- Nerve biopsy will reveal 'onion-bulbs' type nerves from the vicious circle of demyelination/remyelination.
- Genetic testing studies will confirm the defect.

What is the pattern of inheritance?
The most common mutation is in chromosome 17, which encodes the peripheral myelin protein 22. The most common pattern of inheritance of the disease is autosomal dominant.

What are other possible differentials of peripheral sensorimotor neuropathy if it is not hereditary?
Diabetes, alcohol, hypothyroidism, sarcoidosis, vasculitides, paraneoplastic, uraemia, drugs.

> **MNEMONIC**
>
> Other causes of peripheral sensorimotor neuropathy, apart from hereditary.
>
> *DASH-GB*
> **D**iabetes
> **A**lcohol
> **S**arcoid, vasculitides
> **H**ypothyroidism
> **G**uillain–**B**arre/chronic inflammatory demyelinating polyneuropathy (CIDP)

How would you manage this patient?

Supportive treatment with exercise and physiotherapy, walking aids, occupational therapy, orthopaedic surgery, and analgesia for neuropathic pain.

Motor neurone disease

Positive clinical findings

As with a CMT case, the synopsis will be to examine either the lower or upper limbs; however, if you elicit the below findings and have time, try to have a quick look at the opposite (for example, if the guide said to examine the lower limbs, do have a look at the hands as well) to see if the process you have noted in the lower limbs affects equally the upper limbs.

The clinical findings on this case are:

1. proximal and distal wasting with fasciculations, and distal wasting of the small muscles of the hand (sign of lower MND);
2. hypertonia (sign of upper MND);
3. weakness;
4. hyperreflexia, brisk reflexes (sign of upper MND) and
5. sensation is normal.

> **Tip!**
>
> If you have identified limb weakness with intact sensation, but the pattern of MND does not entirely fit with upper motor neurone or lower motor neurone, as there is a combination of both lower and upper neurones, then this is Motor Neurone Disease.

Model presentation

On inspection, the patient has evident bilateral wasting of his lower limbs, distal and proximal, with prominent fasciculations. He has bilateral loss of power in his lower limbs, with a combination of upper and lower motor neurone signs. Sensation is intact. The above combination of findings would be consistent with a diagnosis of MND.

I would like to proceed with examining upper limbs and cranial nerves to identify motor neurone signs elsewhere. I would also like to assess the patient's cognitive function and measure his forced vital capacity to assess whether respiratory muscles are involved in this process.

> **Tip!**
> If on your examination of a case you reveal that there is a sensory deficit, then do not mention MND as part of your differentials! It is a common mistake that candidates make during the exam, and this will not impress the examiners.

Discussion with the examiners

What types of MND are you aware of?
- Amyotrophic lateral sclerosis
- Progressive muscular atrophy
- Primary lateral sclerosis
- Progressive bulbar palsy

How would you investigate this patient?
There are no specific diagnostic tests for MND. Typical clinical findings and excluding other pathologies is the way forward for diagnosing MND. Investigations should start with blood tests, spinal and brain imaging, lumbar puncture for CSF analysis and nerve conduction studies to exclude other diagnoses.
- Electromyography
- Nerve conduction studies
- Neuroimaging
- *Blood tests*: thyroid functions, full blood count, full biochemical profile, serum electrophoresis, autoantibody screen, inflammatory markers
- CSF analysis

How would you manage this patient?

The disease is not curable and management should target control of the patient's symptoms.

Riluzole is one of the agents given to target disease prognosis, but it has not given promising results to date. The prognosis of MND, unfortunately, is not a good one.

Patients need to be managed by a multidisciplinary team and should be educated about their disease. Symptom control should be targeted and individualized to each case.

Myotonic dystrophy

This may be a 'look and approach' case. The synopsis would usually be something that would give away the diagnosis, which is a spot one, and the examination would be focused on revealing the characteristic signs. The guide is usually a general one, such as: 'Look at this patient and examine. His dad died during surgery.'

> **Tip!**
> Once you have made your spot diagnosis of MD, your examination should be focused and systematic, and should aim to demonstrate myotonia. Follow the below order of examination of face and hands.

Face

1. See face (myopathic, expressionless face), take hair off (to assess for frontotemporal balding)
2. Ask to close eyes tightly and open them (to demonstrate myotonia)
3. Check muscle strength in the face (to demonstrate myopathy weakness)

Upper limbs

1. Ask to shake hands
2. Ask to make a fist
3. Formally test for power in upper limbs
4. Tap over thenar eminence

All the above targeted tests will help you demonstrate distal weakness and myotonia.

Positive clinical findings

Face

Myopathic face, frontotemporal balding, ptosis, wasting and weakness of the facial muscles and the sternocleidomastoid. Difficulty opening eyes.

Upper limbs

Distal wasting and weakness and myotonia, with absent reflexes.

Model presentation

On general inspection, this patient has myopathic facies, with frontotemporal balding and bilateral ptosis of his eyelids. There is wasting of his facial muscles, as well as the small muscles of the hands.

On further examination, he has evidence of facial myotonia, as he has difficulty opening his eyes after closure. There is also grip myotonia, as demonstrated by his slow-releasing grip, and percussion over the hypothenar.

I would like to perform a full neurological examination on this patient and then proceed by examining other systems to look for possible complications of the disease.

Discussion with the examiners

What are the possible complications of MD?

- Cardiac
  - arrhythmias
  - heart blocks
  - mitral valve prolapse
  - cardiomyopathy
- Endocrinology
  - diabetes
  - hypogonadism
  - thyroid disease
- Respiratory
  - hypoventilation
  - frequent infections
- Gastrointestinal
  - abdominal pains
  - constipation/diarrhoea

MNEMONIC

Systemic complications of MD: *A-B-C-D-E-F-G-H*

Arrhythmias

Blocks

Cardiomyopathy and mitral valve prolapse

Diabetes and other

Endocrine problems

Frequent chest infections

Gastrointestinal tract disorders

Hypoventilation

How would you diagnose MD?

The diagnosis would be done with a combination of clinical findings, electromyography and genetic testing.

- *Clinical findings*: positive family history and presence of myotonia
- *Electromyography*: for confirmation of myotonia
- *Genetic testing*: useful in confirmation of diagnosis and genetic pattern

What is the pattern of inheritance?

The disease is inherited with an autosomal dominant pattern, and it is caused by a trinucleotide repeat in the myotonin protein kinase gene on chromosome 19.

Parkinson's disease

PD is another one that is a spot diagnosis that you will recognize the moment you get into the room. After you spot the diagnosis, when the guide is general, such as 'this patient has difficulty walking, please examine', you should not waste time being systematic and performing a full neurology examination, as the time will not allow you to finish. You should take advantage of the time given and show the examiners that you know what signs to expect in a patient with PD.

You should concentrate on demonstrating specific signs of PD:

- Ask the patient to walk (characteristic PD gait).
- Ask the patient to close their eyes (blepharoclonus).
- Ask a general question to the patient (monotonous speech).
- Test for cogwheel and lead pipe (wrists and elbows).

- Examine the small movements of the hand (bradykinesia).
- Ask the patient to count backwards from 20, while still examining the upper limbs (signs are exacerbated).
- Ask the patient to write something (micrographia).
- Check for vertical eye gaze (supranuclear palsy).
- Check for cerebellar symptoms (multisystem atrophy).

MNEMONIC

Commands for PD: *WEST Hands*

Walk (to assess posture and gait)

Eyes (for blepharoclonus and gaze)

Speech and writing ('small')

Hands (tremor, rigidity, bradykinesia)

Positive clinical findings

Expressionless face, bradykinesia, slow and monotonous speech, cogwheel rigidity at wrists and lead pipe rigidity at elbows, asymmetrical, coarse, pill-rolling tremor, exacerbated by thought, and less obvious on movement, micrographia, forward-stooping gait, with narrow-based and hesitant steps, and reduced arm swing. Extrapyramidal signs are usually more prominent on one side. Presence of cerebellar or pyramidal signs suggests multisystem atrophy, and vertical gaze palsy suggests progressive supranuclear palsy.

Model presentation

This patient, who presents with a history of falls, has a stooped posture when walking, with narrow-based gait and reduced arm swinging. When his eyes are closed, there is evidence of blepharoclonus. When asked to talk, his speech is monotonous and of low volume. On examination of his upper limbs, there is pill-rolling tremor of the hands and bradykinesia, mostly marked on the right, with lead pipe rigidity of the elbows and cogwheel rigidity of the wrists. The tremor is exacerbated mental activity. The patient's handwriting is typical of micrographia. Eye movements are normal, and there are no cerebellar signs on examination. In summary, this patient has PD. I would like to finish my examination by looking at this patient's observation chart, and specifically looking for postural hypotension and pulse trend as markers of autonomic dysfunction that can contribute to his frequent falls. I would also like to perform a mini-mental test to assess cognitive function.

> **Tip!**
>
> Parkinson-plus syndromes: Differentials to include in your presentation if the following findings are present:
>
> - *Supranuclear palsy*: progressive supranuclear palsy
> - *Low blood pressure in synopsis*: multisystem atrophy

Discussion with the examiners

How would you treat this patient?

What medications are used in the treatment of PD?
- Co-careldopa
- Dopamine agonists (ropinerole)
- Monoaminoxidase inhibitors (selegiline)
- Anticholinergics (procyclidine)
- Apomorphine

How would you investigate this patient?

PD is a clinical diagnosis. Clinical demonstration of bradykinesia in combination with either tremor of rigidity raises the suspicion of PD. Patients presenting as such will have to be referred to a PD clinic, commonly run by either neurologists or geriatric care physicians for further investigations. Brain imaging is usually performed, but the main test for the diagnosis, after clinical suspicion, is the patient's response to dopaminergic agents.

Pattern recognition cases

The other category is the 'pattern recognition/findings'.

For all the below patterns, the most common synopsis would be to examine the patient's lower limbs. That is because the signs will be mainly easily found in the lower limbs; however, if you have identified a specific pattern and you have time left for more examination, then it is advisable that you proceed to examine the upper limbs to determine whether the same process is affecting the upper limbs as well.

> **Tip!**
> Once you recognize a specific pattern, always try to quickly scan the patient for signs that would reveal the underlying diagnosis. Most of them will be there, they will be easy to pick up if you look for them, and the examiners will be impressed!

Cerebellar syndrome

> **Tip!**
> Whenever you are asked to examine the patient's lower limbs, it is a good technique to start by asking the patient to walk for you before you start examining them. Watching their gait and identifying specific gait patterns will make the rest of your examination easy and sleek.

For instance, in this case, if you ask your patient to walk first and notice that they have a broad-based and ataxic gait, you have your diagnosis even before proceeding to the rest of your examination. In this case, you know you will be looking to demonstrate cerebellar signs for the rest of your remaining time.

Positive clinical findings

Gait is broad-based and ataxic. If there is unilateral cerebellar disease, then this would be associated with a tendency to fall to the side of the cerebellar pathology. If the patient is unable to walk without crutches, then observe the way the crutches are held, as they would be broad-based in this case.

Romberg's sign is negative.

The speech is slurred and staccato (ask the patient to say 'baby hippopotamus').

- *Eyes*: there is nystagmus with a fast component on the site of the cerebellar pathology. The saccadic eye movements are abnormal (hypermetric).
- *Upper limbs*: there is dysdiadochokinesis, dysmetria on finger-nose testing and intention tremor (rebound when the eyes are closed).
- *Lower limbs*: there is impaired heel-shin testing, pendular reflexes.

If your patient has cerebellar syndrome, try to identify a cause.

Once you have identified the pattern as bilateral cerebellar syndrome, then proceed to look for quick clues that you can spot within your 6-minute examination that may reveal the underlying diagnosis:

- Demyelination
  - internuclear ophthalmoplegia
- Alcohol
  - chronic liver disease stigmata
- Friedreich's ataxia
  - pyramidal weakness and impaired vibration: dorsal column
- Drug-related
  - medications may be at the side of the patient

If the signs are unilateral, then after presenting your findings, you may want to say to the examiners that you would definitely want brain imaging in the form of MRI to search for cerebellar lesions, vascular or infective aetiology.

Model presentation

This patient has signs of bilateral cerebellar syndrome.

On examination of his upper limbs there is dysdiadochokinesis with intention tremor and dysmetria on finger-nose testing on both limbs, more marked on the right. Similar findings are evident in both lower limbs, as the heel-shin test is impaired in both limbs, more marked on the left.

On walking, the patient adopts a broad-based gait, characteristic of cerebellar syndrome, whilst Romberg's test is negative.

I would like to finish my examination by performing cranial nerve testing, and obtaining a full history, including medication and alcohol history.

MNEMONIC

Causes of cerebellar syndrome: *(DAMN CV)2*

Drugs and metabolic causes
Alcohol and **A**utoimmune
Mitochondrial disorders and **M**imic syndromes (Migraine)
Neoplastic and **N**eurodegenerative
Congenital ataxia
Viruses, **V**itamin deficiency, **V**ascular causes

Discussion with the examiners

How would you investigate this patient?

The first priority in a case like this is to search for a cause that can be reversed by treatment.

- All patients will need brain imaging to exclude obvious causes, and a series of blood tests should be sent.
- Full blood count, full biochemical profile, inflammatory markers and full autoantibody screen, haematinics and thyroid function tests would be the initial screening.
- A full neurological assessment is essential.
- Other tests, such as CSF analysis and more specific blood tests may be needed if the initial screen has failed to reveal a cause.

How would you treat this patient?

The management options will depend on the underlying cause. If the cause is treatable, then this will be the target of treatment; however, if the cause is not reversible, as in most cases, then the patient should be managed via a multidisciplinary approach with supportive treatment for symptomatic control and psychological support.

Peripheral neuropathy

When you are asked to examine a patient's PNS (usually lower limbs), and your findings are bilateral, and symmetrical loss of power suggestive of lower motor neurone type, or bilateral and symmetrical loss of sensation, or a combination of the above, mostly distally, then the underlying pathology that should be mentioned is peripheral neuropathy. If the signs are only motor, then the term you should use is 'peripheral motor neuropathy'. Similarly, if the signs are only sensory, then you should conclude that the patient has an underlying diagnosis of peripheral sensory neuropathy. If the patient has a combination of the above, then the underlying diagnosis is peripheral sensorimotor neuropathy. In this last scenario, you should try to seek other signs that would give away a long-standing process, suggestive of CMT. If so, present your case as CMT disease. If not, then you should mention the general term of peripheral neuropathy, and have CMT as one of your differentials if the signs could be explained by this differential.

Positive clinical findings

Sensory neuropathy

- No motor involvement, no wasting or weakness, reflexes are preserved
- Bilateral sensory loss in a stocking distribution with impairment of light touch, pinprick, vibration and joint position
- Romberg's sign positive
- Ataxia and high-steppage gait

Motor neuropathy

- Distal weakness, of lower motor neurone type, with depressed reflexes, and muscle wasting (distally) if the weakness is long standing.
- Sensation is normal.

Sensorimotor

- Combination of the above

Model presentation

This patient has bilateral and symmetrical weakness of his lower limbs, which is predominantly distal weakness. The weakness is of lower motor neurone type, as the reflexes are suppressed bilaterally, and the plantars are downgoing both sides. There is also wasting of the muscles of his lower limbs. All modalities of sensation are intact, and there are no cerebellar signs on examination. In summary, this patient has peripheral motor neuropathy.

I would like to finish by performing a full neurological examination to see whether this process is affecting the upper limbs as well, and then I would like to take a full history, including drug history.

Discussion with the examiners

How would you investigate this patient?

- This patient definitely needs nerve conduction studies to confirm diagnosis and reveal a pattern of the underlying pathology (demyelinating vs. axonal disease).
- Even before that though, a full history should be obtained, including past medical history, drug history, family and social histories. This point is very important, as it may reveal the possibility of the peripheral neuropathy being part of the symptomatology of a more generalized underlying disease (lymphoma, HIV infection, diabetes, thyroid disease, excess alcohol intake, inflammatory bowel disease, vasculitis, inherited neuropathies).
- Blood tests should be sent for routine investigations, such as full blood count and haematinics, urea and electrolytes, and inflammatory markers, and urine should be sent for protein.
- In addition, more specific blood tests should be carried out, such as serum protein electrophoresis, full autoantibody screen, viral serology for hepatitis viruses, thyroid function tests, HbA1c.
- If the initial tests fail to reveal the underlying diagnosis, then the patient may need to have CSF analysis, spinal MRI, nerve biopsy (CIDP) and genetic testing (CMT).

Spastic paraparesis

The synopsis for this case would be, 'This patient presented with difficult walking. Please examine his lower limbs.'

Positive clinical findings

- Scissor gait; if the weakness is severe, perhaps the patient will not be able to walk at all.
- Pyramidal weakness (with hypertonia, hyperreflexia and extensor plantars).
- Wasting may be present if the weakness is severe and long-standing, or may represent a mixed upper motor and lower motor neurone problem, in which case it falls into the diagnosis of MND.

Once you have identified that there is spastic paraparesis, try to look for possible reasons.
- Mixture of lower motor and upper MND; MND (remember that if there is any kind of sensory loss in the lower limbs, it is bad if you list MND as one of your differentials; MND is purely a motor neurone problem and the examiners will mark you down)
- Sensory level and spinal scar, previous trauma
- Any combination of the 'I COPD' signs of MS; demyelination/MS
- Predominantly dorsal column signs (loss of vibration and proprioception); subacute degeneration of the cord
- Loss of pain and temperature, but vibration and proprioception are intact; syringomyelia (look at the hands)

Tip!

Differential diagnosis of spastic paraparesis and dorsal column signs:

1. MS: look for cerebellar symptoms, optic atrophy
2. Cervical myelopathy lower motor signs in the hands, neck collar
3. Taboparesis Argyll Robertson pupil
4. Friedreich's ataxia cerebellar, pes cavus
5. Subacute degeneration of the cord peripheral neuropathy

Model presentation

This patient has atypical scissors gait on walking. On examination of his lower limbs, there is bilateral symmetrical weakness, with hypertonia and hyperreflexia bilaterally. Both of the plantars are upgoing.

All modalities of sensation are impaired with a level clinically at T8.

There were no cerebellar signs, although the examination in the lower limbs was difficult due to weakness.

In summary, this patient has spastic paraparesis, and it appears that this is due to a lesion in the spinal cord around the level of T8.

> **Tip!**
> 'Paresis' is weakness, 'plegia' is paralysis; do not confuse the terms during the exam. Be specific on your findings. If you find weakness 3/5 and you tell the examiners that the patient has paraplegia, they may think you cannot interpret your examination findings.

Discussion with the examiners

How would you treat this patient?

Multidisciplinary team consisting of physiotherapists, occupational therapists, orthopaedics or neurosurgeons involvement, neurologists and general physicians.

There are treatments available to help with the symptoms of spasticity and pains, but there is not a pharmacological option yet to treat the weakness.

How would you start investigating this patient?

In the first instance, this patient needs a full neurological examination, and spinal imaging in the form of MRI.

Hemiparesis

Positive clinical findings

Upper limb of the affected side: flexor posturing with dystonic posture of the hand.

Lower limb of the affected side: extensor posturing.

Tip!

To observe these findings, it is best to ask the patient to walk. As the patient walks, they will adopt the specific pattern above, and the pyramidal type of weakness of the affected side will become apparent.

- Pyramidal weakness with hypertonia and hyperreflexia on the affected side
- Extensor plantars, Hoffman's sign positive, pronator drift on the affected side
- Hemiplegic circumducting gait

Model presentation

This patient, on walking, adopts a hemiplegic gait on the left, with apparent difficulty on flexing the muscles in his left lower limb, and difficulty on extending the muscles in his left upper limb.

On examination of his lower limbs, there is mild marked hypertonia and hyperreflexia on the left, with weakness on the same side in a pyramidal distribution, with the flexors affected more than the extensors.

The plantar response is upgoing on the left, and there is reduced sensation of all modalities on the same side.

There is also wasting on the left lower limb that probably represents atrophy due to difficulty using this side over the years.

Putting all the above findings together, the patient suffers from left hemiparesis.

I would like to continue with performing a full neurological and cardiovascular examination and taking a detailed history from the patient.

There are no scars on the patient's sculpt, and the patient looks systemically well. I also noted a scar in his neck, which probably represents previous endarterectomy. So the most possible underlying diagnosis would be a previous stroke, which has left the patient with residual weakness.

Discussion with the examiners

What are the possible causes of hemiparesis?
- Stroke is by far the most common cause.
- Other intracranial pathologies that can give rise to unilateral pyramidal weakness are
  - space occupying lesion,
  - trauma,

- previous surgery,
- demyelination and
- localized infection (cerebral abscess).

How would you manage this patient?

The patient's management needs to be in the form of a multidisciplinary approach with organized physiotherapy to try to regain some power in his limbs.

If the patient had an acute ischaemic stroke giving rise to this weakness, then the management needs to be targeted toward prevention of further episodes and reducing cardiovascular risk.

Distal weakness of the upper limbs

Positive clinical findings

Bilateral findings

If the synopsis advises you to examine the patient's hands, and just by a quick scan you notice there is wasting distally in the hands, sparing the proximal upper limbs, then in most cases this represents a central nervous system pathology, as opposed to the opposite; when the weakness is proximal, sparing the distal muscles, then the primary pathology is in the muscle, rather than the central nervous system.

If the distal wasting and weakness of the upper limbs is symmetrical and bilateral, then the possible differentials to be aware of are

- MND
  - normal sensation, combination of upper and lower motor neurone type disease
- syringomyelia
  - loss of pain sensation, but intact joint position and vibration
- cervical myelopathy and
  - sensory loss in specific dermatomes
- peripheral motor (+/− sensory)
  - neuropathy glove distribution and symmetrical

Unilateral findings

- Old poliomyelitis
  - complete weakness/paralysis with normal sensation

- Pancoast tumour or cervical rib
  - sensation loss in dermatomes C8-T1
- Median and ulna palsies
  - relevant nerve distribution

Model presentation

On examination of this patient's upper limbs, there is evident bilateral weakness distally, with wasting of the small muscles of the hands, symmetrically.

There is also sensory loss to all modalities bilaterally, which corresponds to C5, C6 and C7.

I could not elicit the patient's reflexes, despite reinforcement technique.

In summary, this patient has distal symmetrical weakness and wasting of his upper limbs. There is a wide range of differentials that could give rise to wasting and weakness of the small muscles of the hands bilaterally, but given that the patient has sensory loss of all modalities, which corresponds to a specific dermatome distribution, cervical myelopathy would be my top differential.

I would like to perform a full neurological examination of this patient, including examining the lower limbs for spastic paraparesis.

Discussion with the examiners

The questions that may come up are already covered. As you may have noticed, this last pattern is not a new list of neurology diagnosis, but it is a pattern recognition of diseases that have already been explored within this chapter.

Where to find neurology cases to practise

Neurology clinics and stroke wards or neurorehabilitation wards are ideal. Not only will you find a variety of patients, you will also be able to ask for guidance from neurologists on different examination techniques.

Communication and ethics

Introduction

Effective communication skills are integral to the role of a doctor, and so you should look to score highly in this station.

Teaching good communication skills lies outside the remit of this book; however, there are some clinical scenarios that occur frequently in the PACES exam, and there is specific legal, clinical and ethical knowledge required to perform well in these consultations. You need to be familiar with how these issues apply in the United Kingdom.

Often the information you impart to patients in this station is potentially life-changing or highly emotive. Because of this, especially when discussing issues under law, you must be confident, precise and clear with the information and instructions you give.

You must still use structure in this station, much like you would for Station 2. Utilizing a well structured approach will make you appear confident and competent to the examiners, and make you less likely to miss something, get lost or repeat yourself.

It is important that you remain polite, calm and nonjudgmental. If the actor likes you, they are likely to give you more information, and help you if you get stuck.

Although it is important not to patronize the patient, it is important that you do not use technical language or 'jargon'. As doctors, we become so used to using medical terms that we may not even recognize them as such. Practising this station with someone who is not a doctor will help you identify use of technical terms. Alternately if you practise this station with someone with a medical background, instruct them to note when you use jargon. If you find yourself using a technical term like 'biopsy' in the exam, immediately follow this with an explanation to the patient, in this case, 'which is when we take a tiny piece of body tissue to look at under a microscope'.

As with Station 2, it is very important that you ask the patient at some point in the consultation if they have any other concerns. This often reveals important elements to the case you have overlooked, and gives the actor a chance to help you. It also demonstrates empathy and concern for the patient. The best time to do this is just before you summarize your consultation to the patient at the end, along with asking them if they have any other questions. It is also a useful question to ask if you find yourself lost, or if you finish the station early. You must be careful how you phrase this in some circumstances, though; for example, if you are counselling the daughter of a man who was subject of medical error and died, asking, 'do you have any concerns?' will not generate a good response! Instead try more gentle approach; for example, 'is there anything else that concerns or worries you that we haven't talked about so far?'

Always summarize the consultation with the patient and agree on a plan with them before finishing. You may realize that you have missed an important point when doing this, which you can then go back and cover. It also gives the actor a chance to prompt you. It demonstrates to the examiners that you can identify the most pertinent aspects of the consultation in a patient-centred manner. Finally, it allows you to mentally prepare for your presentation to the examiners. Agreeing on a plan with the patient is often an excellent way of checking their understanding of what you have told them. It is also important that you have been explicit in your instructions; for example, you may have told an epileptic patient that they cannot drive, but do they know this must happen immediately and that they cannot drive home?

Remember that the setting for these consultations will normally be on a ward or in a clinic, so you can assume there are resources available to you. You can offer the patient written information, a discussion with a specialist nurse or contact details to support organizations.

The following scenarios have a few examples of frequent encounters in Station 4 of the exam. Although they are specific cases, most of the advice given applies to a wide range of such scenarios that you may come across in the real exam as they contain basic medical ethical principles.

Example scenario 1: DVLA regulations

- *Your role*: You are the core medical trainee year 2 (CMT2) in diabetes clinic.
- *The problem*: Discussion regarding informing the Driver and Vehicle Licensing Agency (DVLA) for medical condition.
- *The patient*: Nicholas Jones, 32-year-old male

Please read the scenario below. When the bell sounds, enter the room. You have 14 minutes for your consultation with the patient, 1 minute to collect your thoughts and 5 minutes for discussion. You may make notes if you wish.

This 32-year-old patient is known to have type 1 diabetes and has been on insulin treatment since he was 16 years old. He has been admitted three times within the last 6 months to the accident and emergency department with hypoglycaemic episodes without warning, and needed urgent treatment. On all three occasions, he was found unresponsive on the street by bystanders and an ambulance was called.

We have gone through his treatment, diet, lifestyle changes and glucose monitoring, and we do not seem to have been able to identify why he has been getting so frequent hypoglycaemias without warning. He is currently monitoring his glucose levels multiple times per day. I have advised him that he should inform the DVLA regarding these episodes, but he would like another medical opinion from his diabetes team.

Your task is to discuss this current problem with the patient, and advise him that he has to inform the DVLA and stop driving until further changes occur with these episodes.

Background

- In the United Kingdom, the DVLA issue driving licences and set out regulations concerning fitness to drive.
- A patient may have a group-1 licence, which includes cars and motorcycles, or a group-2 licence, which includes lorries and buses; the law is different depending on which licence a patient has.

Points to cover in the consultation

- Do not fall into the trap of taking a full medical history, you do not have time and it is not the aim of this station.
- You should take a minute to confirm the diagnosis, ask about current treatment, compliance and glucose monitoring.
- Ask the patient if they have had episodes of hypoglycaemia, and if so how many they have had in the last year. You need to confirm the type of hypoglycaemic episode they are having:
  - Discuss symptomatic hypoglycaemia that the patient is able to correct themselves.
  - Ask about hypoglycaemia without warning (i.e., the patient is only alerted to the hypoglycaemia when performing routing glucose testing).
  - Enquire about hypoglycaemia requiring assistance.
- Take a thorough occupational history. Does the patient rely on driving to make a living? What type of licence do they hold?
- Explore driving within a social context. Do they need to drive to take their children to school?
- Explain to the patient that due to their hypoglycaemia, they should not be driving. Make it clear that this is because of the regulations set out by the DVLA, and not just your professional opinion.

- Tell the patient they should inform the DVLA and stop driving immediately.
- Be prepared for a negative reaction from the patient; they are likely to be angry or upset. Be supportive and empathetic, and give them time to express their feelings. Do not talk over them, become angry or threaten them immediately with breaking confidentiality.
- You can explain that it is for their own safety, the safety of any passengers and the safety of other road users.
- The patient may rely on driving for their job, and may assume that they will lose their job or become unable to support themselves. Again, you must show empathy and stay calm. You might suggest that they could negotiate other duties with their employer.
- Your plan should include reviewing their current insulin regime and lifestyle to try to prevent hypoglycaemic events in the future. You do not need to do this in detail during this consultation, but you should explain to the patient that this will be done in clinic in consultation with them, their diabetes nurse and their GP to develop the regime most suited to them. This allows you to introduce something positive into the consultation, and helps to wrap up the scenario.
- When you summarize and agree on a plan with the patient, you must make sure that the patient knows they should not drive starting from that moment. You should offer them the contact details for the DVLA (you do not need to know these!), and some written information.

Discussion with the examiners

- Driving and diabetes:
  - Group-1 drivers:
    - The patient must inform the DVLA if they take insulin.
    - Their licence will be renewed every 1–3 years.
    - The patient must inform the DVLA and stop driving if they have two or more episodes of hypoglycaemia requiring assistance in 1 year.
    - The patient must inform the DVLA and stop driving if they are hypo-unaware.
  - Group-2 drivers:
    - The patient must inform the DVLA regardless of which medication they take.

- Patients on insulin will need an independent medical assessment every year.
- They will need to regularly record their glucose.
- Hypoglycaemia:
  - Patients are advised not to drive with blood glucose monitoring (BM) less than 4.
  - If patient starts to feel hypoglycaemic while driving, they should pull over to a safe place, take the key out of the ignition, sit in the passenger seat and have some carbohydrate; they should not start driving again for 45 minutes.
- Hypoglycaemia unawareness:
  - Defined as having BM less than 3 with no awareness or symptoms.
- Hypoglycaemia requiring assistance:
  - This is defined as a hypoglycaemic episode where the patient was physically or cognitively dependent on someone else to help them
- Breaking confidentiality to DVLA:
  - If you believe that a patient is unfit to drive, you should tell them so and ask them to inform the DVLA.
  - If the patient will not inform the DVLA and continues to drive, then it is permissible under GMC guidance to break confidentiality and notify the DVLA.
  - Do not say that you would do this; rather, tell the examiners that you would discuss it with your consultant.

Other conditions to be aware of

- Seizure
  - The DLVA mandates that patients with isolated seizure are banned from driving for 6 months, or 1 year if the risk of further seizure is deemed to be greater than 20%.
  - Patients with epilepsy must be seizure-free for 1 year before driving again.
- Obstructive sleep apnoea (OSA)
  - OSA is a common condition that can cause excessive daytime somnolence and lead to patients falling asleep during the day. If it is severe enough, they may be at risk of falling asleep at the wheel.
  - If patients with OSA are sleepy during the day, they must inform the DLVA. This is the same for any condition causing daytime sleepiness.

- Acute coronary syndrome
  - Patients treated with angioplasty must abstain from driving for 1 week.
  - Patients not treated with angioplasty must not drive for 4 weeks.
- Visual problems
  - Drivers must be able to read a licence plate at 20 m, and their visual acuity must be 6/12 on a Snellen chart.
  - If patients wear glasses or contact lenses, then they should wear these when assessing their capability to drive.

Further tips for this type of scenario

These rules may change with time, so make sure you visit the DVLA website before sitting your exam, in order to be up-to-date with the current rules.

Example scenario 2: Breaking bad news

- *Your role*: You are the CMT2 in the respiratory clinic.
- *The problem*: Breaking bad news
- *The patient*: Jason Horton, 56-year-old male

This patient has been complaining of cough and shortness of breath for a few months. A recent chest X-ray was arranged by his GP and revealed a shadow that warranted further investigations. A recent CT revealed metastatic lung cancer. The patient has been referred to the lung cancer multidisciplinary team (MDT). In the meanwhile, a 2-week referral had been arranged before the CT scan and you are the doctor in clinic, meeting this gentleman for the first time.

Your task is to inform the patient of the diagnosis and advise on further plan.

Background

- Breaking bad news is a common scenario for a PACES exam. It is also a scenario that is common in a doctor's day-to-day practice and you will be expected to perform well.
- This scenario relies less on specialist or legal knowledge, with an emphasis on sensitive and compassionate communication.

Points to cover

- Introduce yourself and ensure the patient is comfortable. Check the patient's identity. You should always do this; however, it is especially important in this consultation.

- You must be in a position where you can make good eye contact and effectively pick up on nonverbal cues as these are vital in this scenario.
- Ask if there is anyone with them today; you will demonstrate to the examiner that you are aware of how important social support will be for this patient.
- Starting with a brief open question such as 'how are you today?' allows you to establish some rapport, and may provide a clue as to how the actor may react to the news; they may mention they are anxious about the results of their scan.
- Briefly recap events to date; this will smoothly lead you into discussing the diagnosis. For example, 'I understand that your GP referred you to our clinic because you have been short of breath and have coughed up some blood, so we have requested a scan to see if we can find out what is causing the problem'.
- Do not fall into the trap of taking the medical history again. This is not the focus of the consultation and it may look like you are delaying breaking the news. The patient likely knows that they are here for the scan results, and may become impatient and interrupt you.
- Signal that you are going to discuss the scan results.
- Use a 'warning shot'. This is a single sentence to prepare the patient for bad news; for example, 'the scan has shown something quite serious', or 'I'm afraid I don't have good news'. This is not an opportunity to delay breaking the bad news, or try to push the patient into guessing the diagnosis.
- You should pause briefly between the warning shot and the diagnosis, but not long enough that the patient feels the need to interrupt or request the diagnosis.
- State the diagnosis clearly and concisely without medical jargon.
- Use the word cancer. It must be said at least once, otherwise your communication may not be clear. Avoid medical words such as 'tumour', vague terms such as 'mass' or euphemisms such as 'a shadow on the lung'.
- Once again, pause. This will allow the patient to take in the information and allow them to set the agenda for the next portion of the interview.
- If after an appropriate pause the patient does not speak, ask an open question to invite them to share their feelings and initial reaction; for example, 'News like this can be a very big shock, and I expect there are a lot of things going through your head at the moment. What would you like to discuss?'

- Expect a very emotional response and for the patient to go through several reactions before they are ready to receive further information and make a plan.

- Patients may start with denial and ask if you are sure about the diagnosis, or sure that it is their scan. This is why it is important to check their identity at the beginning of the conversation; now is not the time to check their name and date of birth.

- After the initial denial, the patient may become angry. Remember they are not angry at you, so avoid becoming defensive. Keep calm and continue to give information in a clear and concise way.

- The patient may then ask how long they have to live, or if the cancer is treatable. Unless you have been given specific information in the briefing, avoid getting into specifics. This can be an ideal time to now move forward to the plan.

- Check that the patient is ready to move on. They may indicate this by asking what the next step is, or you could ask them, 'Do you want to talk about what we need to do next?'

- In this scenario, further investigations are required to arrive at a firm diagnosis. Briefly outline the investigations. Unless you are specifically instructed to in the introduction, you do not have time to explain what a positron emission tomography scan is, or consent for a bronchoscopy.

- In other scenarios, the next appropriate step may be MDT discussion or urgent referral to oncology.

- Allow the patient the opportunity to ask questions about the plan.

- Invite the patient again to express any concerns or particular feelings they have right now. The patient may have a specific concern that you must address in the scenario, such as fear of dying in pain, or how they will tell their spouse.

- Recap the plan, and check the patient's understanding. This is signalling that you are coming to the end of the scenario.

- How you finish the consultation is vital. Patients with cancer diagnoses often feel isolated and scared. Before you end the scenario, you must discuss the support available and the immediate plan.

- In clinical practice, this is often when the Macmillan nursing team or specialist cancer nurse will become involved. You can explain to the patient that the nurse will also see them now, discuss any further questions they may have and give them contact numbers and written information.

Discussion with the examiners

- Referral to cancer services
  - Under NICE guidance, referral for suspected cancer is an 'urgent' referral, and patient should be seen within 2 weeks. This is often referred to as a '2-week wait referral'.
  - Treatment for cancer must start within 31 days of the decision to treat, and within 62 days of the initial referral.
- The role of the MDT in the diagnosis of cancer
  - NICE recommends that cancer diagnosis and treatment decisions should be made through an MDT.
  - The makeup of MDTs vary in different specialties and hospitals, but normally consist of specialty consultants, radiologists, histopathologists and specialist cancer nurses.
  - The MDT process offers multiple advantages.
    - Accurate diagnosis and staging
    - Treatment decisions are made after discussion among multiple specialists
    - Improved continuity of care
    - Better adherence to national guidelines
    - Improved access to clinical trials
    - Good communication among primary, secondary and tertiary care
    - Efficient use of resources
    - Patient-centred care with patients offered the information and support they need.

Other scenarios to be aware of

- Other life-changing diagnoses:
  - HIV or other bloodborne viruses:
    - Be aware of the social stigma that may accompany these diagnoses.
    - Older patients may remember the 'tombstone campaign' of the 1980s, which portrayed HIV as a terrifying fatal disease and they may not be aware that HIV is a treatable condition, and they could have a near-normal life span.
    - You may need to address transmission to/from partners.
  - Neurological disease such as multiple sclerosis or motor neuron disease:

- These are often progressive diseases, and conveying this without denying the patient hope requires a careful balance.
- Remember not to overload patients with information about these often complex neurological diseases. Now is not the time to show off your knowledge of pathophysiology to the examiner. Keep the consultation patient-centred.
- Death of a relative:
  - Breaking bad news should follow a similar structure with appropriate use of pauses and warning shots.

Further tips for this type of scenario

- Although there are good communication models to use for breaking bad news such as the Cambridge-Calgary model, there is no single script that will guarantee success in these scenarios.
- It is important to practise these scenarios as much as possible so you can develop skills in reading nonverbal communication and the use of pauses.
- Role playing as the patient with a colleague can be a good way of improving your skills. This is a very patient-centred scenario and you should have an idea of what the patient is thinking throughout. Being on the receiving end of 'pauses' can help you understand when they are useful and how long they should be.
- Imagine how you would like a doctor to speak to one of your relatives if they were alone and receiving bad news.
- When appropriate, try to accompany experienced senior colleagues when they are breaking bad news in clinical scenarios.

Example scenario 3: Confidentiality case

- *Your role*: You are the CMT2 in the genitourinary medicine (GUM) clinic.
- *The problem*: Discussion over HIV status disclosure.
- *The patient*: Daniel King, 37-year-old male who has recently been diagnosed with HIV infection.

You are the SHO in the GUM clinic. This patient has been diagnosed with HIV. He has been refusing to disclose this information to his partner. Your task is to convince the patient that he needs to disclose and discuss the above diagnosis with his partner or any sexual contacts.

Background

- Confidentiality is a key principle in patient care; however, there are a few highly specific situations in which it may be necessary to breach patient confidentiality.
- Although treatable, HIV infection causes fear amongst patients and can carry significant social stigma, which inhibits patients from disclosing their status.

Points to cover

- Introduce yourself and enquire how the patient is feeling. You should attempt to quickly establish rapport.
- How you approach the case will depend on the scenario background. If another healthcare professional has expressed concerns, then you should gently lead up to the discussion by making social enquiries and asking if he currently has a partner.
- After asking about the partner and how the relationship is progressing, you could then ask if he has discussed his HIV status.
- Ask if he is sexually active, and if so, ask if he is practising safe sex.
- You could now open the discussion and ask the patient if he has thought about disclosing his diagnosis, and what his fears may be.
- You should offer to support the patient in disclosing his diagnosis either by discussing how he may approach this, or by offering to see him and his partner in clinic together.
- You should advise the patient on safe-sex practice.
- You should state that the patient is putting his partner at risk of HIV transmission and potentially delaying his diagnosis and treatment.
- If the patient still does not wish to disclose his diagnosis to his partner, you should explain that in certain rare cases, a doctor may breach confidentiality to inform an individual who is at risk.
- You should advise them that reckless transmission of HIV is a criminal offence under United Kingdom law.
- You must then re-enter discussion with the patient, and support him in finding a way to disclose his diagnosis to his partner. If he does not feel able to do this immediately and needs time to think, it is important to arrange followup in a few days so this can be discussed again. Advise him to practise safe sex by using a condom or abstain from sex until he has discussed this with his partner.
- Conclude by asking the patient if he has any other worries or questions.

Discussion with the examiners

- Reckless transmission of HIV:
  - Reckless transmission of HIV is a criminal offence under United Kingdom law subject to a maximum sentence of 5 years per individual infected.
  - The criteria for reckless transmission are met if the individual has unprotected sex with someone who does not know they have HIV, if the individual is aware they have HIV and understands how HIV is transmitted, and that their sexual partner can contract HIV.
  - Reckless transmission is not the same as intentional transmission, which is a malicious and intentional act to transmit the disease.
- A medical professional may disclose HIV status when there is a serious, identifiable risk to a specific individual who would be at risk of transmission if not informed. It is essential that the patient is counselled and supported to inform their partner before then, and they must be informed that you intend to breach confidentiality. The decision should be made by a senior member of a specialist team, such as a GUM or infectious disease (ID) consultant.
- Barriers to HIV disclosure:
  - Patients with HIV and AIDS still experience discrimination from some sections of society.
  - Although it spread awareness of HIV, the tombstone campaign in the United Kingdom in the 1980s has been attributed to spreading fear of the diagnosis of HIV.
  - Many people still do not know that HIV is a treatable disease or how it is transmitted.
  - Fear of social stigma and the perception that HIV is a rapidly progressing fatal disease inhibits patients from seeking HIV testing.
- When can a doctor break confidentiality?
  - Contacting the DVLA if a patient continues to drive against medical advice
  - Informing the police of gunshot and knife wounds when failure to disclosure would put the patient or another individual at risk, or if disclosure may help in the prevention, detection or prosecution of a serious crime
  - Other serious notifiable diseases
  - Disclosing the name and address of a patient when required to do so under the Road Traffic Act of 1988

Other scenarios to be aware of

- Taking consent for HIV testing
- Counselling an individual for postexposure prophylaxis
- Patients with OSA, epilepsy or hypoglycaemia who should not be driving
- The police requesting information about a patient
- A colleague with a drug or alcohol problem.

Further tips for this type of scenario

- Breaching confidentiality is always a final option once all others have been explored. Leave discussion of this once you have exhaustively explored all other options with the patient.
- Do not give the opinion that you are threatening or blackmailing the patient with the potential to breach confidentiality.
- Remember that you would require to have a successful ongoing therapeutic relationship with this patient, and for them to disengage with services would be disastrous for them, as well as their partner.
- Practise discussing sexual partners and taking sexual histories if you do not already have expedience for clinical practice. It is important you do not feel awkward asking these sensitive questions in front of the examiners.
- When in stations dealing with HIV issues, do not make assumptions about sexuality. Be aware that some men who have sex with men may be in long-term stable relationships with women, do not identify as 'gay' or homosexual and so will deny this if asked.
- Patients should always be informed if you are planning to breach confidentiality.
- Often decisions are made if they are 'in the public interest'. Reading some case studies should give you a good feel for how this is determined.
- You should never make this decision in isolation. Make sure you mention in the discussion that you would involve at minimum your consultant and possibly also the MDT, a second opinion or your medical defence organization for advice (remember you would not disclose any personal information to your medical defence organization).
- If possible, speak to a GUM or ID specialist about how they have approached these situations in the past.

Example scenario 4: Communicating a medical error to patients

- *You are*: The CMT2 covering the elderly ward.
- *The problem*: Communicating a medical error to patient/relatives
- *The surrogate*: Miss Louise Williams, daughter of Darren Williams, 87-year-old male in the elderly ward

This 87-year-old man on your ward, who was admitted with pneumonia, has been prescribed the wrong dose of diuretic and subsequently developed acute renal failure. Your task is to discuss this with his daughter, who wishes to make a complaint.

Background

- Up to 10% of hospital inpatients in the United Kingdom experience some sort of adverse event, and many of these are medication errors.
- It is important to be honest and upfront when discussing errors with patients and their families. The national health service (NHS) promotes an open approach to discussing medical error.

Points to cover

- Introduce yourself and explain your role. Confirm who you are speaking with and their relationship to the patient.
- A patient or relative in this type of scenario is likely to be angry and may have a lot to say; allow them time to talk uninterrupted. Do no talk over them or interject.
- Open with an apology, and acknowledgement of the error. Repeat her key concerns to show that you have listened to them. Explain that you would like to talk through what happened, discuss her concerns and then explain what will happen next.
- You will be given the clinical background and events leading up to the error. Explain this in full to the relative. You should fully disclose what happened and not make light of the error or its consequences.
- Do not be tempted to hide behind medical terminology. Not only does it demonstrate poor communication skills to use terms the patient's relative will not understand, it may also appear that you are trying to avoid explaining what happened.
- When discussing the error, do not apportion blame. You may think you know from the scenario who was at fault (the nurse for giving the wrong medication, or the foundation year-1 doctor for writing the wrong

medication on the drug card), but in reality there are often multiple failures that result in an error.

- The patient's relative may have already decided who is at fault in this scenario and may ask you to support their assumption. Again, it is important not to blame any individuals at this stage, but do not anger the relative by disagreeing with them directly. Stating that you cannot comment as you do not have all the facts or were not there but that there will be a full investigation, acknowledges their opinion and your position without contradicting them.

- It is important that you fully explore the consequences of the error, but also discuss how these complications are being, or will be, managed. This avoids painting an overly bleak picture and also shows you are taking a proactive approach in managing them.

- Once you have explained the error, its consequences and how you will manage these, ask if the relative has any questions and is ready to move on. You should now discuss incidence reporting and investigation.

- Explain that a critical incident form will be completed, and then the cause of the error will be investigated. You should also mention who you have notified, which at a minimum should be the consultant in charge of the patient's care. You should explain that the purpose of the incident reporting and investigation is to establish exactly how the error happened, and how to stop it from happening again.

- The relative may still wish to make a complaint. If they do, after your discussion, offer to provide them with the contact details of your hospital's department that deals with complaints. This may be called PALS (patient advice and liaison team), PST (patient support team) or PET (patient experience team), and they will support them in making a complaint. You can also offer to arrange a meeting with the consultant in charge of the patient's care.

- As always, you should draw the station to a close by briefly summarizing the conversation and plan, and asking the patient's relative if they have any other questions or concerns. You can again apologize for the error.

Discussion with the examiners

- Actions following a medical error:
  - Recognition and immediate management.
  - Good documentation of what has happened. This will aid the investigation and follows good practice for open reporting of incidents.

- Approaching the patient and their family to openly apologize for the error. This should be comprised of an acknowledgement and explanation of the error, an apology and explanation of the investigation process.
- Reporting the incident in line with local trust policy. There is usually a standard 'incident form', which can be completed by anyone documenting the error, harm caused and the immediate plan.
- Isolated issues or themes are identified on a local and national scale and are used to amend guidelines or issue safety alerts to prevent the error happening again.
- Dealing with complaints from patients and their relatives.
- Patient safety in the NHS:
  - The patient safety domain of NHS England supports the identification of, understanding of and management of risk to patient safety. This has replaced the National Patient Safety Agency.
  - Incident reports are managed by the National Reporting and Learning System.
  - Key areas targeted by the patient safety domain include fall prevention, preventing pressure ulcers and preventing avoidable venous thromboembolism.

Other scenarios to be aware of

- You may have to discuss an error with the patient or their relatives.
- Common errors include:
  - Delay in diagnosis caused by missing signs or not following up test reports.
  - Incorrect medication administration leading to end-organ damage.
  - Medication being administered that the patient has a documented allergy to.
- Although not strictly errors, some scenarios may be approached in a similar manner, or may be perceived by patients as an error:
  - Recognized complication to an intervention such as lumen perforation in endoscopy. This may be contributed to by failure to follow guidelines for correct procedure.
  - Recognized side effects of medication such as liver injury caused by anti-TB therapy. This may be contributed to by failure to monitor the patient as prescribed by guidelines.

- Haemorrhage caused by anticoagulant or antiplatelet therapy.
- Postponement of investigations or management.
- Anaphylactic reactions to drugs (when allergy unknown) or adverse reaction to blood products.
- Healthcare-acquired infections.

Further tips for this type of scenario

- Apologize early and often. Apology is not an admission of guilt.
- Medical defence organizations report that one of the leading causes of complaints against doctors is a failure to communicate with patients and their relatives.
- Patients making complaints after a medical error often report that what they wanted was someone to listen to them, openly explain what was happening and an assurance that steps were taken to ensure the error did not happen again.
- The aim of the station is not to persuade the relative not to make a complaint. If after your explanation they still wish to make a complaint, help them as much as possible with this. Know what your local patient liaison team is called and how they will support the patient so you can use this in the exam. This will vary slightly from hospital to hospital and the PACES centre will not expect you to know their individual local policy.
- Avoid becoming defensive or contradicting the patient's relative.
- Do not criticize a colleague's actions.

Example scenario 5: Capacity and action against medical advice

- *Your role*: You are the CMT2 in the general medical ward.
- *The problem*: Communication with patient who wants to self-discharge.
- *The patient*: Mrs Julie Lorry, 48-year-old female.

You have been called to the ward to talk to a 48-year-old lady who is being treated for urosepsis and wishes to self-discharge. This lady was admitted overnight, and has been receiving intravenous antibiotics. The consultant reviewed her in the morning in the ward round, and has documented that she needs at least 48 more hours of intravenous antibiotics, with daily bloods and medical review to decide whether she can be safely changed to oral antibiotics.

Your task is to explain to the patient that it is not safe for her to go home before completing the consultant's management plan.

▸ Example scenario 5: Capacity and action against medical advice

Background

- Patients self-discharge for a number of reasons, and if they have the capacity to make the decision, they cannot be compelled to stay (except in certain IDs as specified by the Health Protection [Part 2A orders] Regulations 2010).
- It is important to ensure the patient has the capacity to take their own discharge, and that the best possible care in the situation is provided for them.

Points to cover

- Introduce yourself and explain to the patient why you are here.
- Ask the patient in an open and nonconfrontational way what issues they have encountered.
- The patient may have multiple reasons why they wish to leave. Give them time to talk about them all, and then explore them individually.
- State your understanding of the diagnosis and treatment plan. Explain the reasoning behind the current treatment and need to stay. The plan may not have been conveyed to the patient, or they may be feeling better after initial treatment and not understand why they still need to stay. In this case, the patient may not understand why they need intravenous antibiotics when they have previously had tablets for 'water infections', or understand the importance of waiting for blood cultures.
- Explain the risks of leaving now. You should not try to scare the patient; starting with 'you could get sepsis and ultimately die' will damage rapport and she is likely to disengage with you and is less likely to be convinced by what you say. Start with the most likely consequence, 'you may get high fevers again and feel more unwell', and then move on to the more serious sequelae.
- Explore each of the patient's concerns in turn, and try to find a solution to each. For example, if the ward is too noisy for the patient to sleep, then you could discuss trying to find a side room.
- Some concerns may be outside your control, such as childcare and employment issues. In these cases, you should explore these with the patient and ask if there is any possibility for support from family or negotiation with employers.
- The patient may then decide to stay. In this case, you should then ask if there is anything else that they would like to discuss, or have not

covered. You should summarize her concerns, the agreed upon solution and the immediate action plan.

- If the patient still wishes to leave, then you should negotiate a plan that provides them the best management available in the safest way. In this example, you may offer the patient a course of oral antibiotics. You could ask them if they could return to the ward for a review and repeat blood tests, or offer to make an appointment with their GP in a few days for a checkup.

- It is important you provide an appropriate 'safety net'. This should include important warning signs that they are becoming more unwell. In this example, it may be high fevers, back pain and passing little or no urine. You must also explain to them what they should do if they get these symptoms or feel more unwell. This could include contacting their GP, NHS 111, dialling 999 or returning to A&E. Stress that they can still return to the hospital and seek further treatment even though they have taken their own discharge.

- You should explain to them that they will need to sign paperwork confirming that you have discussed these issues with them, that they understand the risks, know what to do if they become unwell and are legally willing to accept the consequences of this. Approach this gently; do not give the impression that this form is to ensure you do not get in trouble.

- During the consultation, you should assess the patient for capacity. A patient may only take their own discharge if they have the capacity to do so.

- Checking the patient understands the situation and what you have told them demonstrates good communication skills and also assesses an aspect of capacity.

- You should politely ask them to repeat back to you the risks and plan you have communicated to them. You could put this as, 'Could I ask you to run through what I've said so I can ensure I've explained everything well enough?'

Discussion with the examiners

- The Mental Capacity Act of 2005 sets down the criteria for assessing a patient's capacity:
  - You should start with a presumption of capacity, and support the right of the individual to make their own decision. Patients have the right to make unwise decisions.

‣ Example scenario 5: Capacity and action against medical advice

- You should act in the best interest of patients deemed to lack capacity and utilize the least restrictive intervention.
- An individual is deemed to have capacity when they are able to:
  - understand the information needed to make the decision
  - retain that information
  - use that information as part of the process of making the decision; and
  - communicate their decision by verbal or nonverbal means.
- A capacity assessment only applies to one decision and is time-sensitive. A patient may lack capacity because of delirium but improve with treatment, or a patient may lack the capacity to decide their discharge destination but retain capacity to make decisions around their treatment.
- The Health Protection (Part 2A orders) Regulations 2010 can allow a patient to be detained in hospital or other suitable environment to protect others from infection. This applies to specific diseases, and a very specific set criteria must be met to enforce this.

Other scenarios to be aware of

- Patients with mental health problems and unrelated medical illness:
  - The Mental Health Act states that patients under section can only be treated against their wishes for psychiatric problems, and not psychical problems unless the psychical disorder is related to the mental disorder as a symptom or underlying diagnosis.
- Explaining why patients need to stay for investigations, e.g. a computed tomographic pulmonary angiography (CTPA) or lumbar puncture (LP).
- Patients wishing to self-discharge who have an ID specified in the Health Protection Regulations.

Further tips for this type of scenario

- Do not argue with the patient, do not try to frighten them or adopt a dismissive approach.
- Do not mention the discharge against medical advice form until you are approaching the end of the scenario. Some patients see it (as they do consent forms) as an easy way for doctors to absolved themselves from responsibility.

- Remember in a PACES scenario you can assume you have resources that may not normally be readily available to you in day-to-day practice, such as side rooms or alternative options for catering.
- If the patient still decides to self-discharge, this does not mean you have failed the station. It may be that this is how the scenario is scripted to run.
- A good safety net is essential. Make sure you allow yourself time to discuss this fully.
- Completing a discharge against medical advice form is not a legal requirement, but is good practice to document the conversation you have had with the patient.

Brief clinical consultations

Introduction to Station 5

Although Station 5 is a common fear amongst candidates, it really is your opportunity to compensate for any losses from any other station, as what you are asked to do is exactly what you do in your everyday life while on the acute medical unit, with the only difference being the diagnosis is easier to spot and more straightforward than in real life. Thus, you should consider Station 5 the easiest of all as it involves tasks you are more familiar with. So, do approach it as an opportunity to gather marks and perhaps compensate for losses in other stations.

Station 5 has two cases. There are 5 minutes of preparation time for both cases.

You spend 10 minutes with each patient. This is split into 8 minutes of focused history, examination and discussion with the patient, and 2 minutes of discussion with the examiners. Before your 8 minutes with the patient comes to an end, you will get a 1-minute warning from the examiners.

Passing Station 5

Achieving full marks in Station 5 can be 'life saving' in the PACES exam. This is for two reasons:
- It carries the most marks compared with any other station.
- It allows you to display competency in all the different domains on the examiners' mark sheet.

Because Station 5 used to be a 'spot diagnosis' station, these patients are still in the examiners' pool for exams and commonly appear in Station 5. These patients are often those with endocrine, musculoskeletal, eye and dermatological problems.

Other patients included in Station 5 will be those with commonly encountered acute pathology that will be easy to diagnose with a combination of a focused history and focused examination.

The last category of encounters in Station 5 are the surrogates. Those are professional actors who do not in reality have any specific clinical pathology, but a scenario is scripted for them, and they are acting as standardized patients.

In this chapter, we will present some example cases along with a proposed way to approach any case in Station 5 to help you organize your performance and perfect your presentation in the exam.

Presentation technique

Before the start of Station 5, you are given the scenarios, pencils and papers for notes, and 5 minutes to prepare for the cases.

When you read each case prior to the station, from the description of the case and the symptoms mentioned in the scenario, write down a provisional list of differential diagnoses.

> **Tip!**
> In the 5 minutes before entering Station 5, you have to prepare both scenarios as you will not be given time in between cases! Make sure you utilize your time appropriately.

Everybody approaches Station 5 in a different way. Try to practise many cases in your acute medical unit so you can identify your own way of approaching Station 5. It is essential that you develop a technique that works for you and then use this strategy during the exam.

I am going to propose the way that has worked for me, and for the candidates I have been teaching, but remember this station tests how a doctor would act in real-world encounters, and each one of us has a unique way of approaching cases and a unique way of working. So there is not a standardized pattern that works for every candidate.

Proposed strategy

For each scenario, create a flowchart with differentials and subsequently elements in the history and examination that will help you identify the correct diagnosis amongst the differentials you have thought of.

Within the flow chart, write down all the questions you may want to ask the patient regarding each differential to direct you toward the correct diagnosis.

At the same time, make a list of focused examination elements that you need to include to help you confirm each differential.

When you enter the station, try to identify in your preparation period what works better for you. Some doctors prefer to simultaneously ask the questions they have written down, and clinically examine the patient at the same time. Others prefer to take a history first and then examine the patient. No matter which way you prefer, remember that you only have 8 minutes for both history and examination, including a short discussion with the patient about their condition, so you should practise a lot on how to be focused on the information you have to elicit and the examinations you have to perform within the consultation. Do not spend time asking unnecessary questions and performing examinations that will not help you with establishing a diagnosis.

This way, you will be able to eliminate some of the differentials quickly, allowing you to focus your examination to reach one of your suspected diagnoses.

Some of the cases in Station 5 will be more straightforward, and even reading the scenario will lead you to suspect the diagnosis. In these cases, you only have to prepare your focused questions and examination for one diagnosis.

Please see the generic example below with the above proposal technique applied.

Station 5 scenario example

This is the template you will be presented with in Station 5 of the PACES exam:

Clinical problem: This lady is attending the general medical outpatient clinic complaining of...

Physiological observations for the patient above	Reading on arrival
Respiratory rate (respirations per minute)	16
Pulse rate (beats per minute)	120
Systolic blood pressure (mm Hg)	110
Diastolic blood pressure (mm Hg)	70
Oxygen saturations (%)	98% OA
Temperature (°C)	Apyrexial
Other relevant observation data (units if applicable)	

Your task is to:

- Assess the problem by means of a brief focused clinical history and a relevant physical examination. You do not need to complete the history before carrying out the appropriate examination.
- Advise the patient of your probable diagnosis (or differential diagnoses), and your plan for investigation and treatment where appropriate.
- Respond directly to any specific questions/concerns the patient may have.

Example template on note keeping in preparation of the clinical encounters of Station 5:

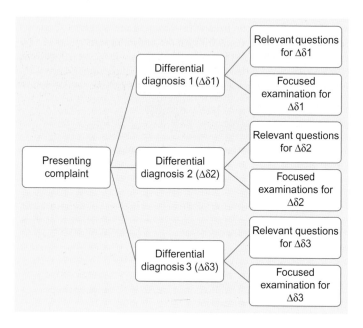

You would start by asking the questions above and performing the suggested targeted examinations. Try to put your differentials in an appropriate order, with the first differential being your most suspected correct diagnosis from the information given in the scenario. If you confirm clinically your first listed diagnosis, you will not need to go any further with all the questions and examinations of your flowchart, but instead concentrate more on examining in more detail for the condition you suspect the patient has.

After that, you might want to ask your patient about relevant past and family medical histories and ask about medication history. This is not a history-taking station, and you will not be marked down if your questioning or examination technique is not structured.

When the examiners inform you that you have 2 minutes left with your patient, start explaining to patient in a couple of lines (and not more), what you think is going on to give rise to their symptoms, and ask them if they have any particular concerns.

> **Tip!**
> Never forget to explain your diagnosis to your patient and explore their concerns. These two elements are worth 4 marks in this station, and they are extremely easy to achieve!
>
> Getting unsatisfactory by both examiners in both cases in 'managing patient's concerns' in Station 5 can make you fail the whole exam!

Case 1: Practical example of above strategy

Clinical problem: Please see this patient who presented with a neck lump.

Physiological observations for the patient above	Reading on arrival
Respiratory rate (respirations per minute)	22
Pulse rate (beats per minute)	110
Systolic blood pressure (mm Hg)	150
Diastolic blood pressure (mm Hg)	80
Oxygen saturations (%)	96
Temperature (°C)	36.6

Your task is to:

- Assess the problem by means of a brief focused clinical history and a relevant physical examination. You do not need to complete the history before carrying out the appropriate examination.
- Advise the patient of your probable diagnosis (or differential diagnoses), and your plan for investigation and treatment where appropriate.
- Respond directly to any specific questions/concerns the patient may have.

▶ Case 1: Practical example of above strategy

Your differentials at this point from reading the scenario would include thyroid goitre or lymphadenopathy. (Of course there are many more differentials of a neck lump, such as hyoid bone, thyroglossal cyst, branchial cyst, carotid aneurysm and many others, but you have to be remember this is a medical exam, so ENT cases will not come up.)

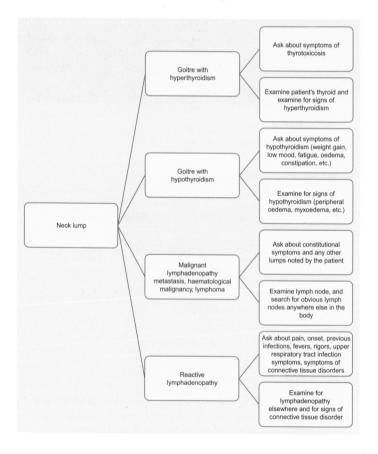

On the initial opening question of the presenting complaint, more often than not, the patient will have to volunteer some of the above symptoms to you, in most cases, enough to make you suspect the first differential of the above table. For instance, if on this example the patient volunteers on initial questioning that they felt occasional palpitations and noticed they were losing weight despite their appetite being increased, hence why they sought medical help, and the doctor then noticed a lump and referred them to you, hyperthyroidism should therefore be your first differential, and you should mostly concentrate on questioning and examining for proving hyperthyroidism symptoms and signs.

Hyperthyroidism

Focused questions to ask if hyperthyroidism is suspected

- Sweaty hands?
- Pins and needles in hands?
- Diplopia?
- Palpitations?
- Chest pains?
- Diarrhoea?
- Weight loss?
- Heat intolerance?
- Leg rashes/skin changes?

Signs of hyperthyroidism on focused examination

- *Hands*: tremor, sweaty palms, tachycardia, atrial fibrillation
- *Eyes*: lid lag, exophthalmos, mixed ophthalmoplegia
- *Legs*: proximal myopathy, pretibial myxedema
- *Neck/thyroid*: palpate for goitre, auscultate for bruit.

Hyperthyroidism biochemically

- TSH low, low end of normal
- T3/T4 raised
- Antithyroid peroxidase (TPO) antibodies positive in Graves and Hashimoto
- AntiTSH receptor stimulating antibodies (TRAb) positive in Graves (specific for Graves)
- Ultrasound thyroid.

Causes of hyperthyroidism
- Graves
- Thyroiditis (Hashimoto, deQuervain)
- Single toxic adenoma
- Toxic multinodular goitre
- Struma ovari
- Drug-induced (iodine, amiodarone, thyroxine).

Treatment of Graves
Antithyroid drugs (ATD): carbimazole, propylthiouracil
- ATD titration
- Block and replace therapy
- Radio-iodine treatment (not in pregnancy, teenagers or thyroid eye disease)
- Surgery.

Treatment of toxic multinodular goitre
Radio-iodine therapy
In a nutshell

Cases in Station 5 can be any presenting complaint with any combination of signs. It can include any pathology you come across in the acute medical unit when on call; however, as Station 5 used to test specific specialty cases in the past, hospitals hosting the exams may still have a pool of patients who used to participate for this station, so it is still common for patients in Station 5 to have an underlying diagnosis of the following:

1. Endocrinology
2. Dermatology
3. Ophthalmology
4. Rheumatology.

Part of your preparation should be to practise on common presentations of:
- Pituitary problems, such as acromegaly and hypopituitarism
- Thyroid disease, hyperthyroidism and hypothyroidism
- Adrenal problems, like Cushing's and Addison's
- Diabetes, with all its complications
- Skin rashes
- Systemic diseases associated with characteristic skin lesions

- Visual problems and diseases diagnosed on fundoscopy, such as diabetic and hypertensive retinopathy, retinal vein and artery occlusion, retinitis pigmentosa
- Rheumatoid arthritis
- Systemic lupus erythematosus
- Psoriatic arthropathy
- Scleroderma

Practical example cases

The following cases are examples of brief clinical consultation scenarios, so you may become familiar with the format of the new Station 5. Try to practise in groups of two or three and time yourselves until you achieve completing a full brief clinical consultation case in 8 minutes without missing important questions and tests.

Scenario 1: Headache

Clinical problem: This 40-year-old lady is attending the acute medical unit with new onset headache.

Physiological observations for the patient above	Reading on arrival
Respiratory rate (respirations per minute)	16
Pulse rate (beats per minute)	90
Systolic blood pressure (mm Hg)	140
Diastolic blood pressure (mm Hg)	90
Oxygen saturations (%)	98% OA
Temperature (°C)	Apyrexial

Your task is to:

- Assess the problem by means of a brief focused clinical history and a relevant physical examination. You do not need to complete the history before carrying out the appropriate examination.
- Advise the patient of your probable diagnosis (or differential diagnoses), and your plan for investigation and treatment where appropriate.
- Respond directly to any specific questions/concerns the patient may have.

▸ Case 1: Practical example of above strategy

Scenario 2: Arthritis

Clinical problem: Please see this lady who has been referred by her GP with pain in her hands and joints.

Physiological observations for the patient above	Reading on arrival
Respiratory rate (respirations per minute)	16
Pulse rate (beats per minute)	70
Systolic blood pressure (mm Hg)	130
Diastolic blood pressure (mm Hg)	75
Oxygen saturations (%)	98
Temperature (°C)	36.6

Your task is to:

- Assess the problem by means of a brief focused clinical history and a relevant physical examination. You do not need to complete the history before carrying out the appropriate examination.
- Advise the patient of your probable diagnosis (or differential diagnoses), and your plan for investigation and treatment where appropriate.
- Respond directly to any specific questions/concerns the patient may have.

Scenario 3: Palpitations

Clinical problem: Please see this 72-year-old lady who has presented to the acute medical admissions unit with palpitations.

Physiological observations for the patient above	Reading on arrival
Respiratory rate (respirations per minute)	22
Pulse rate (beats per minute)	110
Systolic blood pressure (mm Hg)	150
Diastolic blood pressure (mm Hg)	80
Oxygen saturations (%)	96
Temperature (°C)	36.6

Your task is to:

- Assess the problem by means of a brief focused clinical history and a relevant physical examination. You do not need to complete the history before carrying out the appropriate examination.
- Advise the patient of your probable diagnosis (or differential diagnoses), and your plan for investigation and treatment where appropriate.
- Respond directly to any specific questions/concerns the patient may have.

Scenario 4: Shortness of breath

Clinical problem: Please assess this 60-year-old lady, who has a long history of asbestos exposure and has presented with shortness of breath on exertion since 3 months ago.

Physiological observations for the patient above	Reading on arrival
Respiratory rate (respirations per minute)	20
Pulse rate (beats per minute)	90
Systolic blood pressure (mm Hg)	150
Diastolic blood pressure (mm Hg)	80
Oxygen saturations (%)	94
Temperature (°C)	36.6

Your task is to:

- Assess the problem by means of a brief focused clinical history and a relevant physical examination. You do not need to complete the history before carrying out the appropriate examination.
- Advise the patient of your probable diagnosis (or differential diagnoses), and your plan for investigation and treatment where appropriate.
- Respond directly to any specific questions/concerns the patient may have.

Scenario 5: Chest pain

Clinical problem: Please see this 64-year-old male who has presented to the general medical unit with frequent episodes of chest pain on exertion.

Physiological observations for the patient above	Reading on arrival
Respiratory rate (respirations per minute)	16
Pulse rate (beats per minute)	80
Systolic blood pressure (mm Hg)	160
Diastolic blood pressure (mm Hg)	80
Oxygen saturations (%)	98
Temperature (°C)	36.6

Your task is to:

- Assess the problem by means of a brief focused clinical history and a relevant physical examination. You do not need to complete the history before carrying out the appropriate examination.
- Advise the patient of your probable diagnosis (or differential diagnoses), and your plan for investigation and treatment where appropriate.
- Respond directly to any specific questions/concerns the patient may have.

Scenario 6: Loss of vision

Clinical problem: Please see this 72-year-old lady who has presented to the acute medical admissions unit with acute loss of vision in her right eye.

She has a past medical history of diabetes, hypertension and previous TIA.

Physiological observations for the patient above	Reading on arrival
Respiratory rate (respirations per minute)	18
Pulse rate (beats per minute)	110
Systolic blood pressure (mm Hg)	170
Diastolic blood pressure (mm Hg)	80
Oxygen saturations (%)	97
Temperature (°C)	36.6

Your task is to:

- Assess the problem by means of a brief focused clinical history and a relevant physical examination. You do not need to complete the history before carrying out the appropriate examination.
- Advise the patient of your probable diagnosis (or differential diagnoses), and your plan for investigation and treatment where appropriate.
- Respond directly to any specific questions/concerns the patient may have.

Scenario 7: Swollen calf

Clinical problem: Please see this 52-year-old patient who has presented to the acute medical admissions unit with a history of pain and swelling in his right calf.

He suffers from osteoarthritis of his knees and hips, and recently had an elective total hip replacement.

Physiological observations for the patient above	Reading on arrival
Respiratory rate (respirations per minute)	22
Pulse rate (beats per minute)	110
Systolic blood pressure (mm Hg)	150
Diastolic blood pressure (mm Hg)	80
Oxygen saturations (%)	96
Temperature (°C)	36.6

Your task is to:

- Assess the problem by means of a brief focused clinical history and a relevant physical examination. You do not need to complete the history before carrying out the appropriate examination.
- Advise the patient of your probable diagnosis (or differential diagnoses), and your plan for investigation and treatment where appropriate.
- Respond directly to any specific questions/concerns the patient may have.

Scenario 8: Skin rash

Clinical problem: Please see this 22-year-old lady who presented to the general medical outpatient's department with a history of facial rash.

She has a past medical history of unprovoked deep vein thrombosis in her right leg, and a couple of miscarriages in the past.

She is on warfarin and PRN analgesia.

Physiological observations for the patient above	Reading on arrival
Respiratory rate (respirations per minute)	22
Pulse rate (beats per minute)	110
Systolic blood pressure (mm Hg)	150
Diastolic blood pressure (mm Hg)	80
Oxygen saturations (%)	96
Temperature (°C)	36.6

Your task is to:

- Assess the problem by means of a brief focused clinical history and a relevant physical examination. You do not need to complete the history before carrying out the appropriate examination.
- Advise the patient of your probable diagnosis (or differential diagnoses), and your plan for investigation and treatment where appropriate.
- Respond directly to any specific questions/concerns the patient may have.

Index

Note: Page numbers followed by *b* indicate boxes, *f* indicate figures and *t* indicate tables.